Getting Ready for My Doctor's Visit

A Going to the Doctor Book for Kids

This book belongs to:

Written by Dr. Fei Zheng-Ward   Illustrated by Moch. Fajar Shobaru

Copyright © 2024 Fei Zheng-Ward

All rights reserved. Published by Fei Zheng-Ward, an imprint of FZWbooks. No part of this book may be copied, reproduced, recorded, transmitted, or stored by any means or in any form, electronic or mechanical, without obtaining prior written permission from the copyright owner.

Identifiers: ISBN 979-8-89318-040-4 (eBook)
              ISBN 979-8-89318-039-8 (paperback)
              ISBN 979-8-89318-090-9 (hardcover)

A doctor is specially trained to help you feel better when you are sick and enjoys seeing you stay healthy and strong.

You can see the doctor even when you're feeling well.

Grown-ups go to their doctors, too.

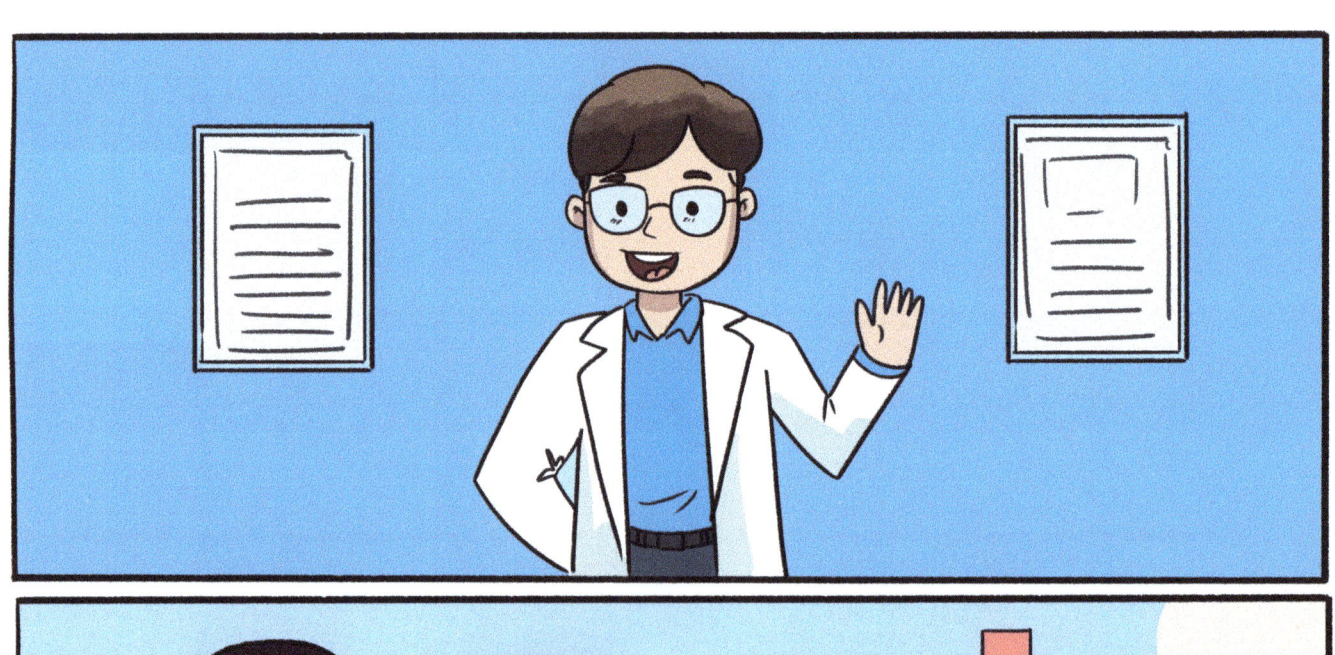

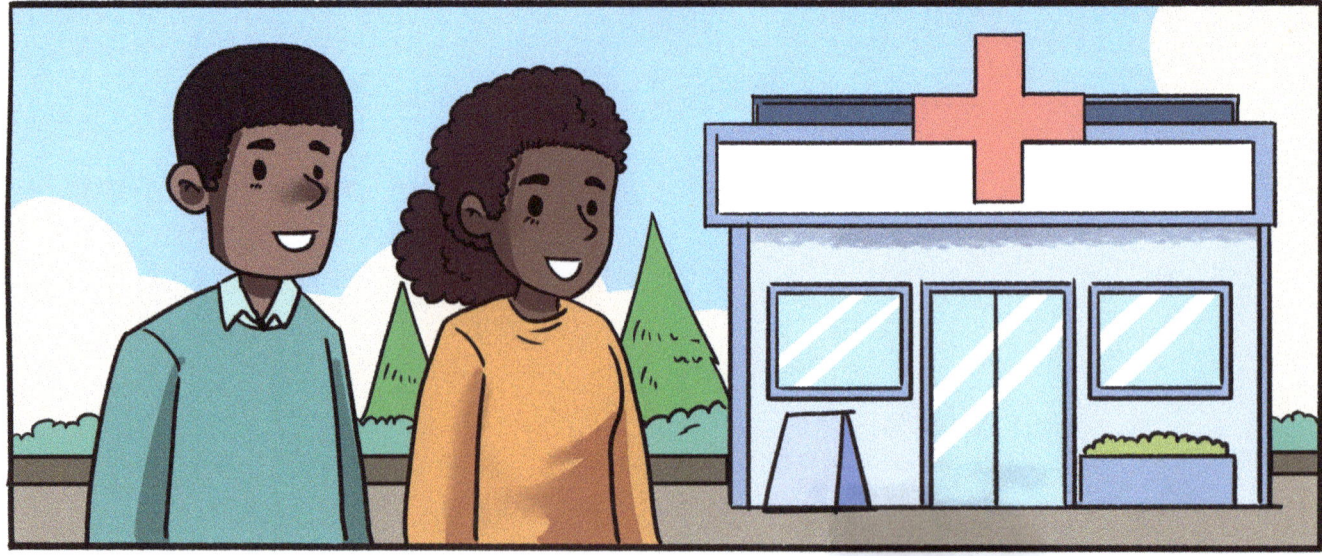

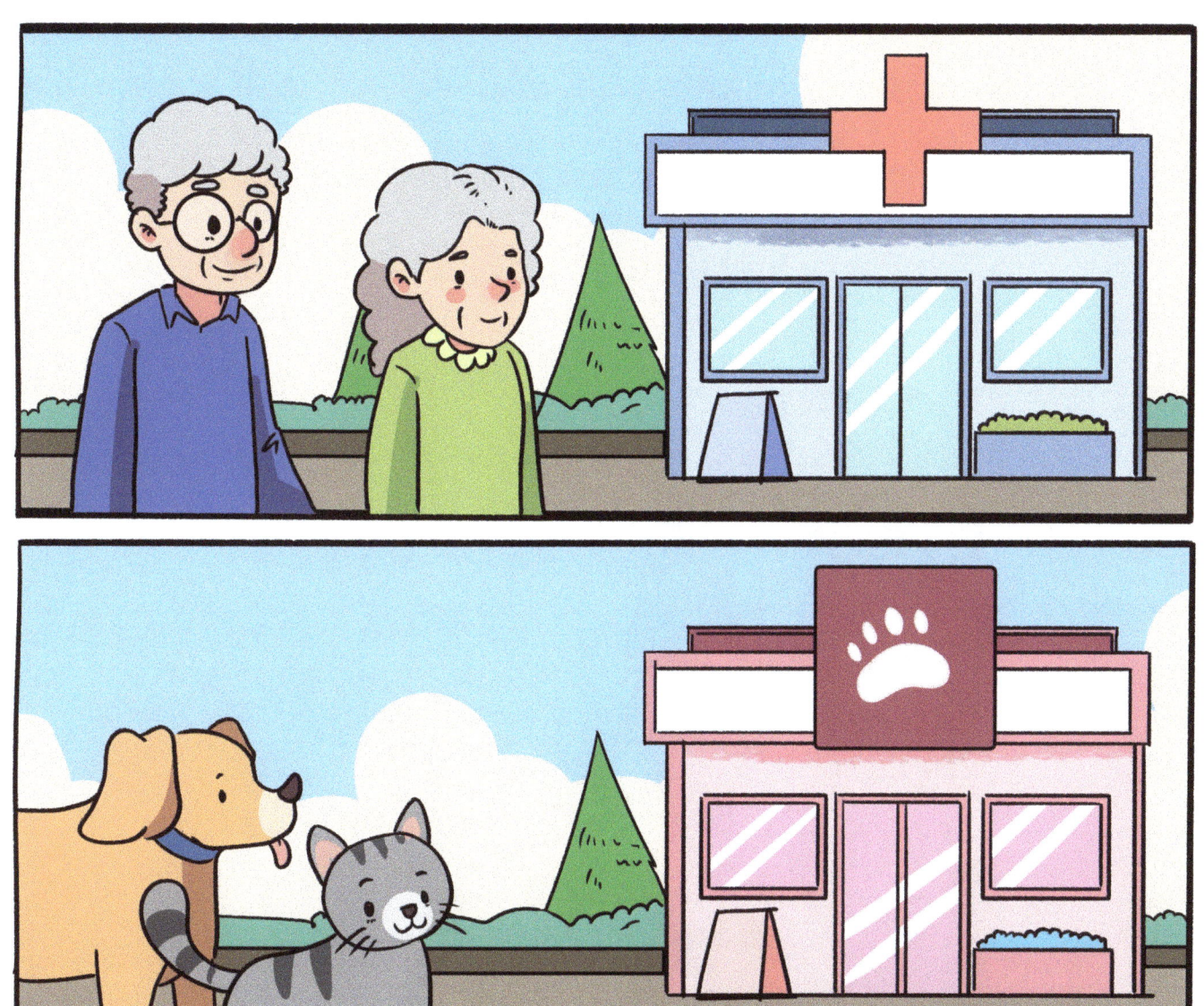

Did you know that dogs and cats go to their doctor, known as a veterinarian (vet), as well?

Have you been to a doctor before?

Circle your answer: Yes or No

On the day of your doctor's visit, you will arrive at their office.

You can bring your favorite toy or blanket.

You may feel a little nervous; that's OK.

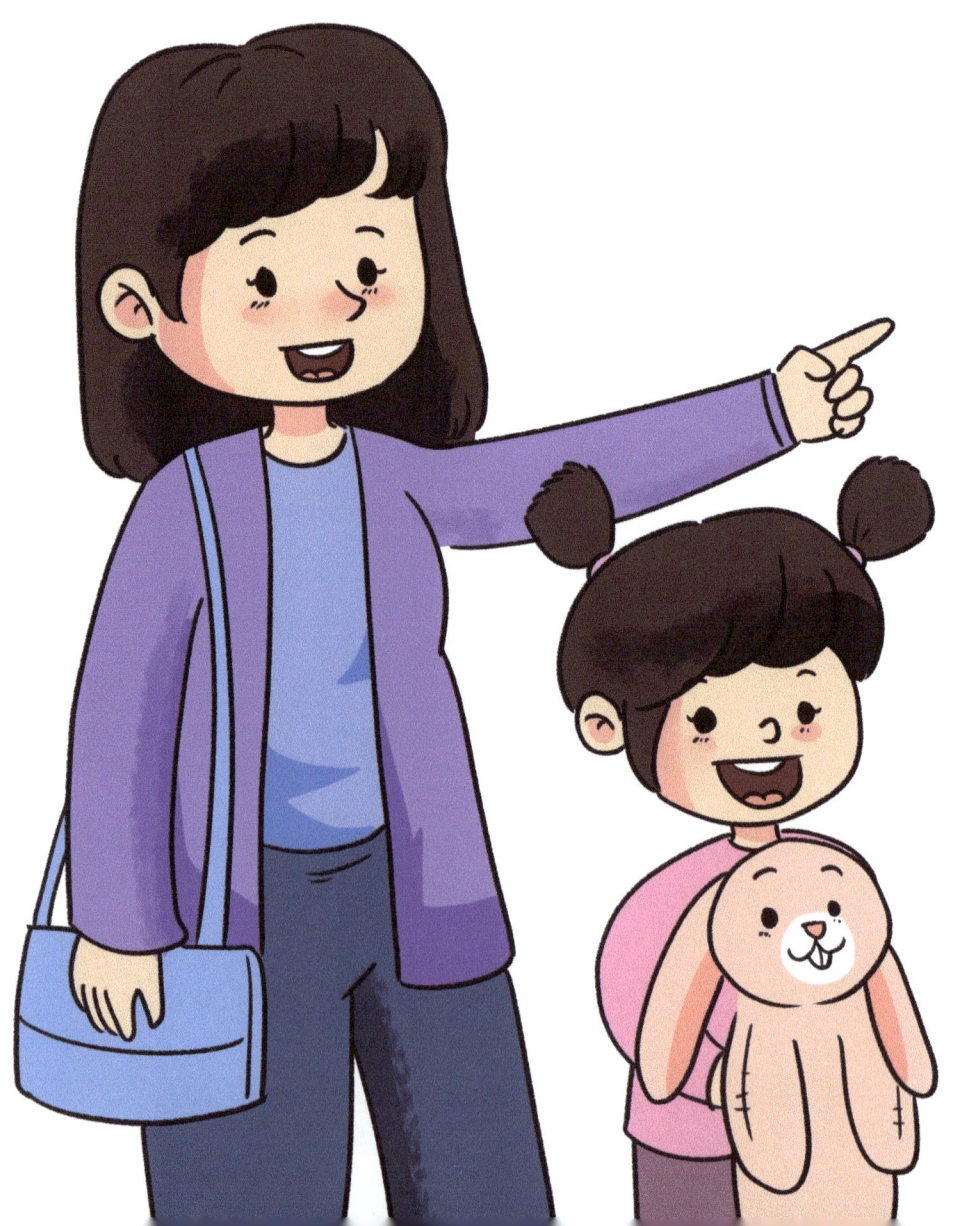

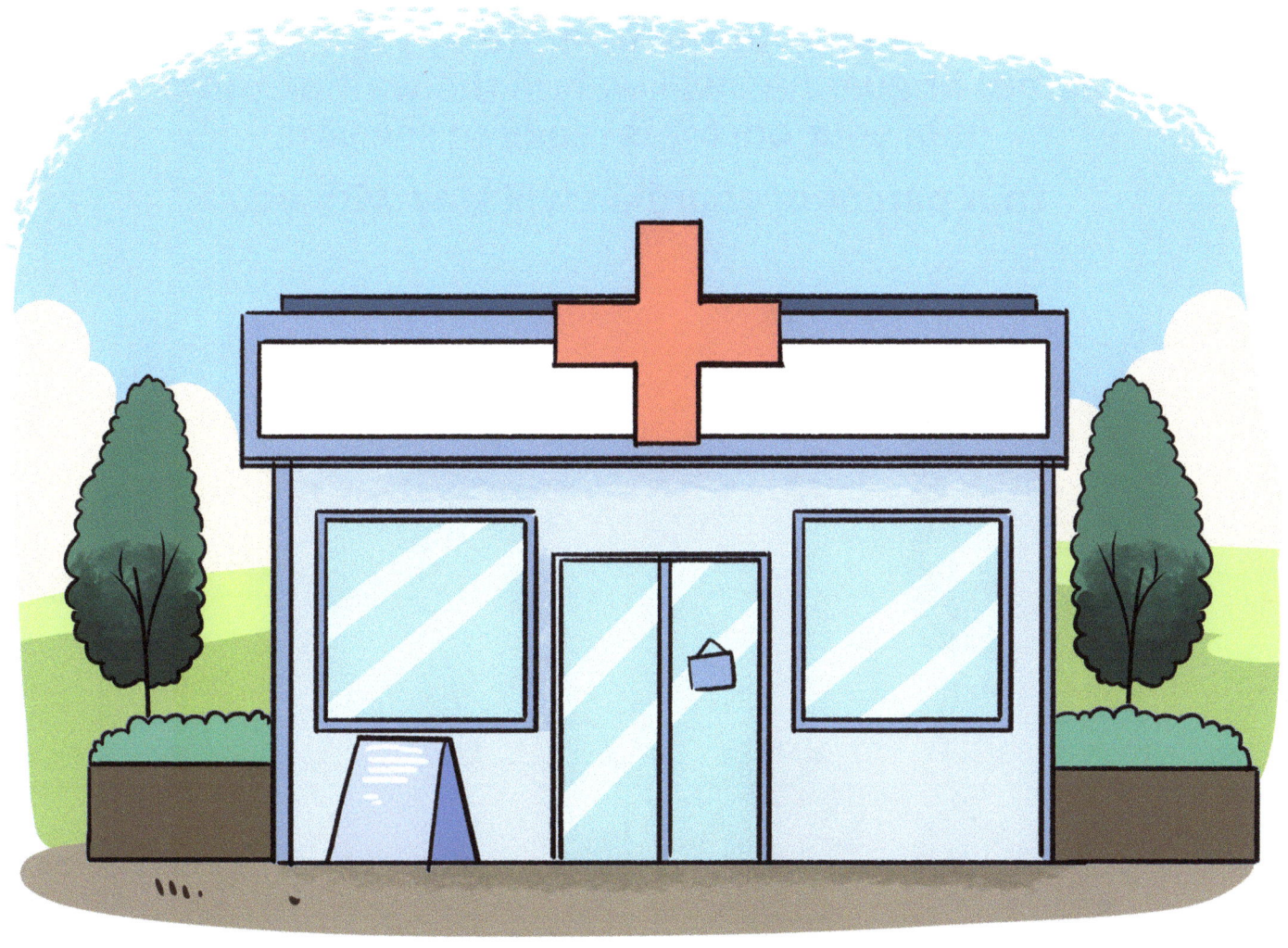

What do you plan to bring with you?

Write your answer here:

_____

After checking in at the front desk, you and your parent or guardian will wait in the waiting room until your doctor is ready to see you.

Your parent or guardian will stay with you.

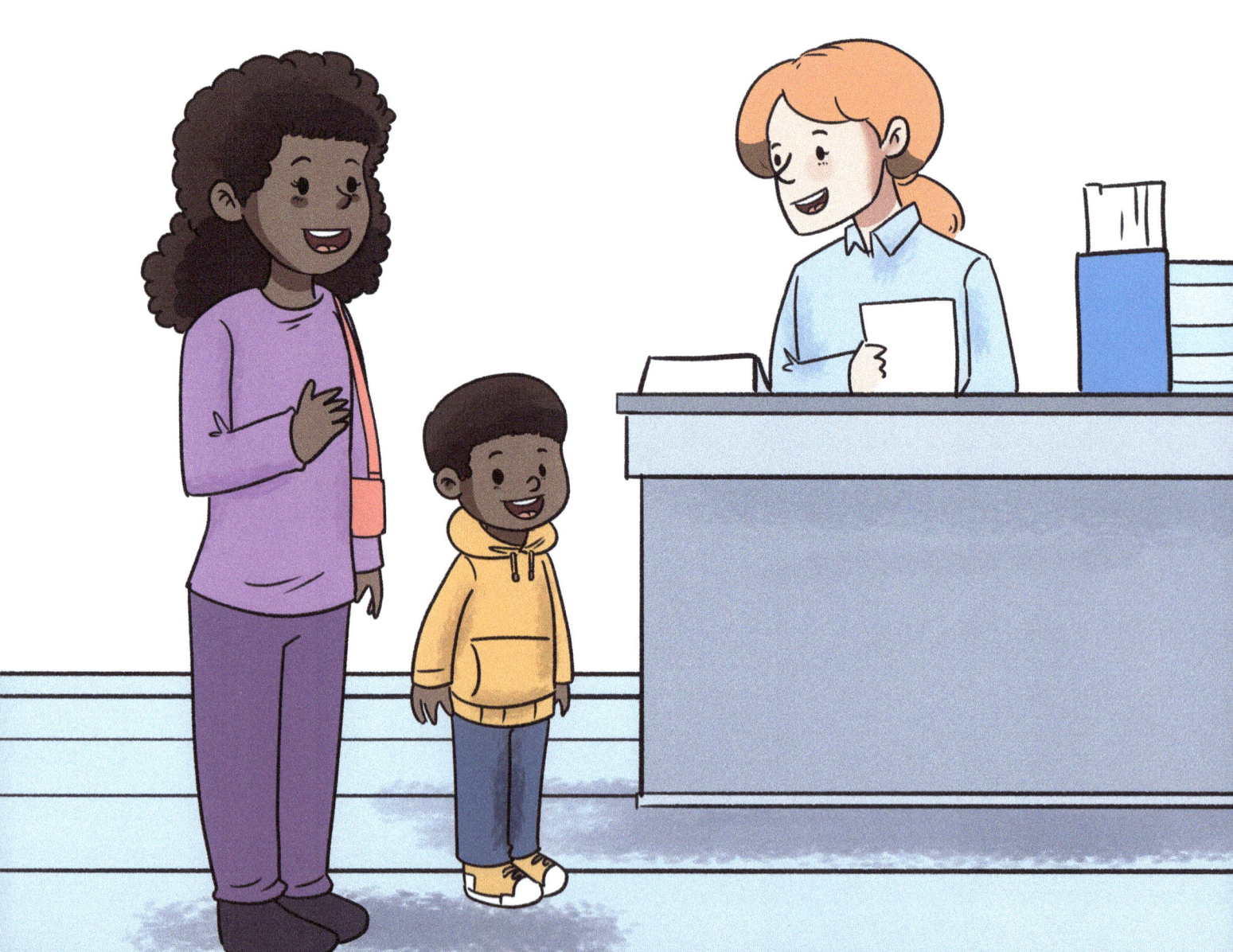

_____, you've got this!
(Write your name here)

Everyone is here to cheer you on!

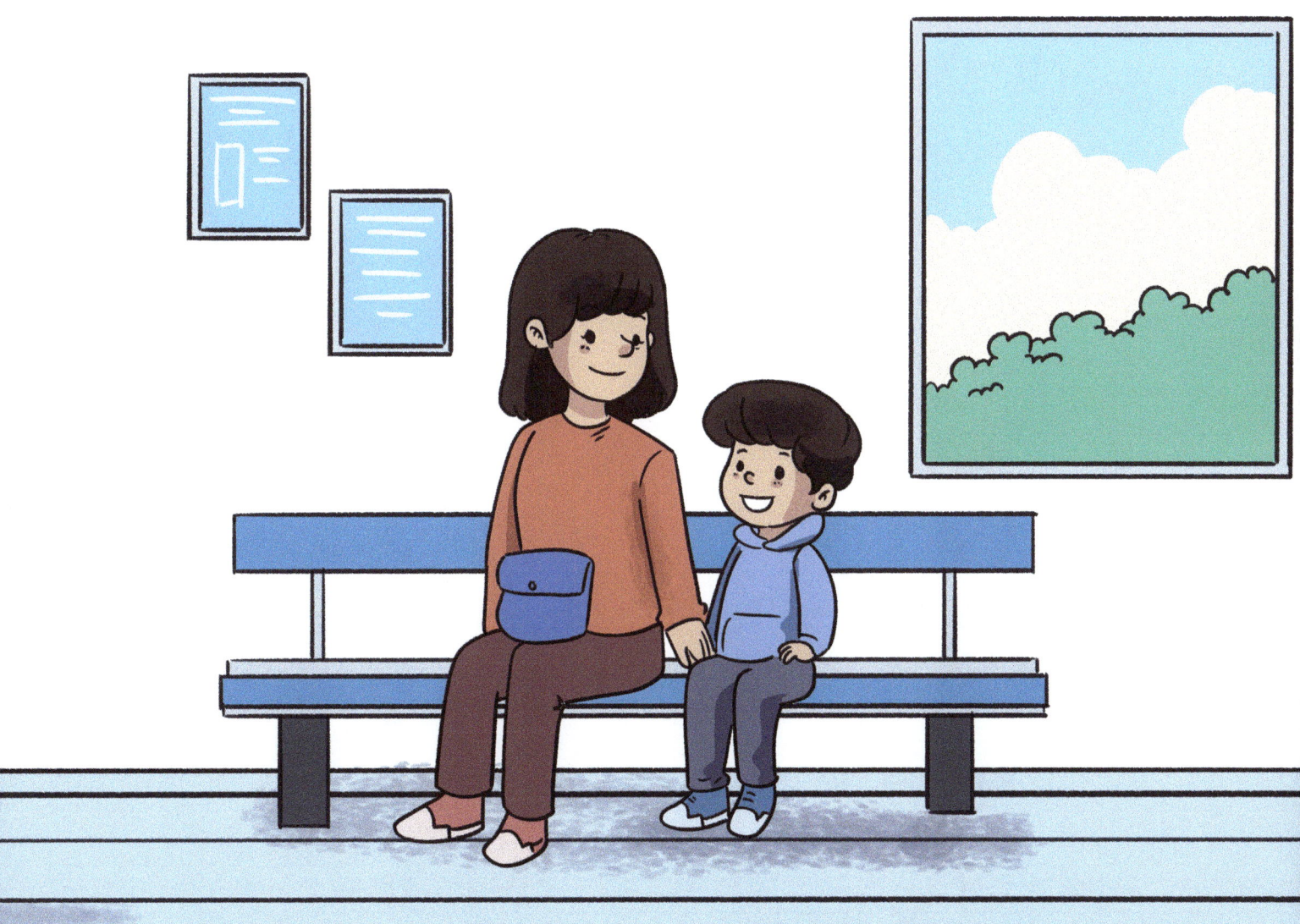

Your nurse, your doctor's helper, will check your weight and height before you see your doctor.
Do you know how much you weigh?
Do you know how tall you are?

My weight is:

_____

My height is:

_____

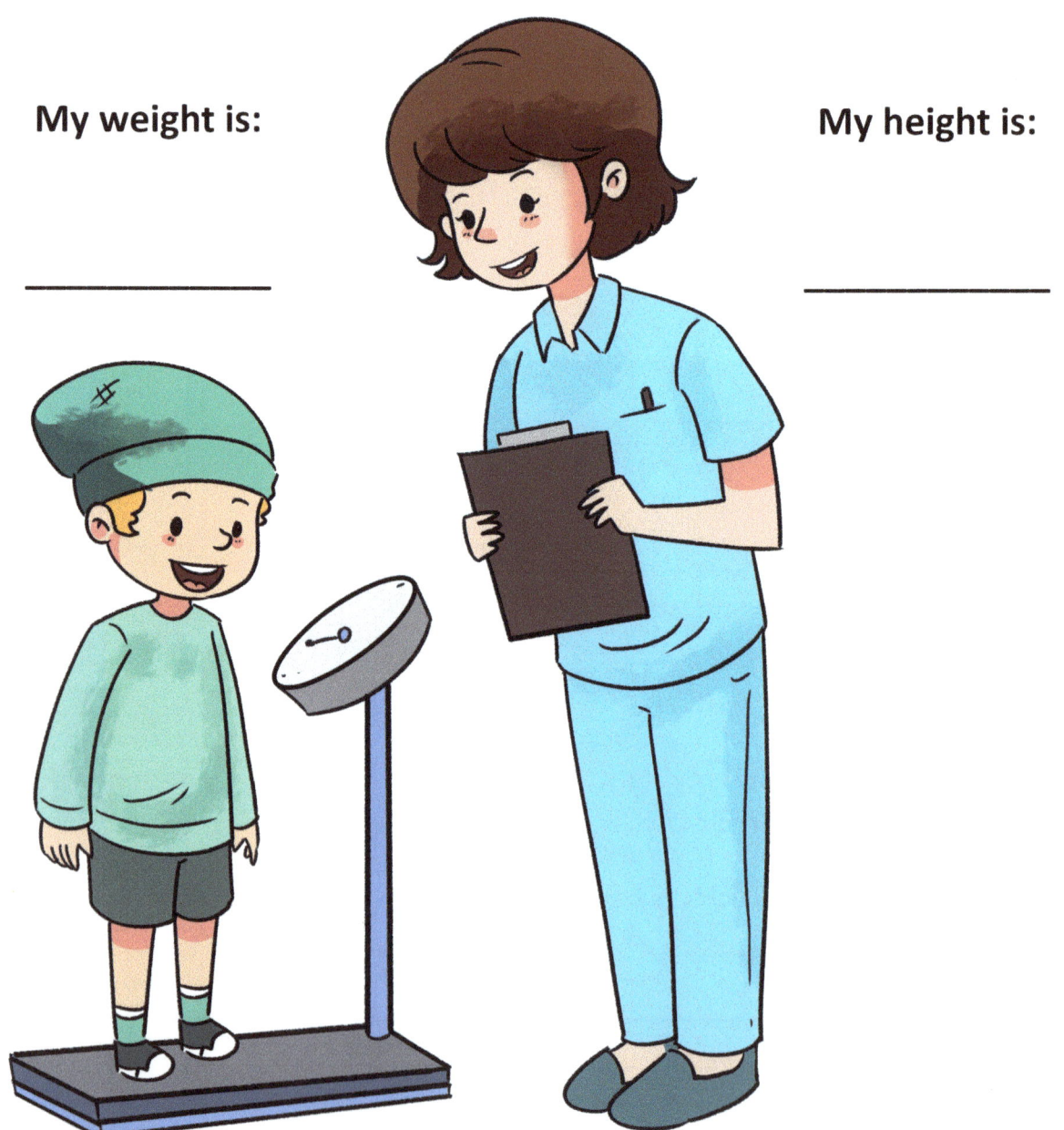

You will get a blood pressure cuff around your arm.

The cuff will give you a BIG squeeze.

Don't forget to stay still while they're examining you.

Are you ready?

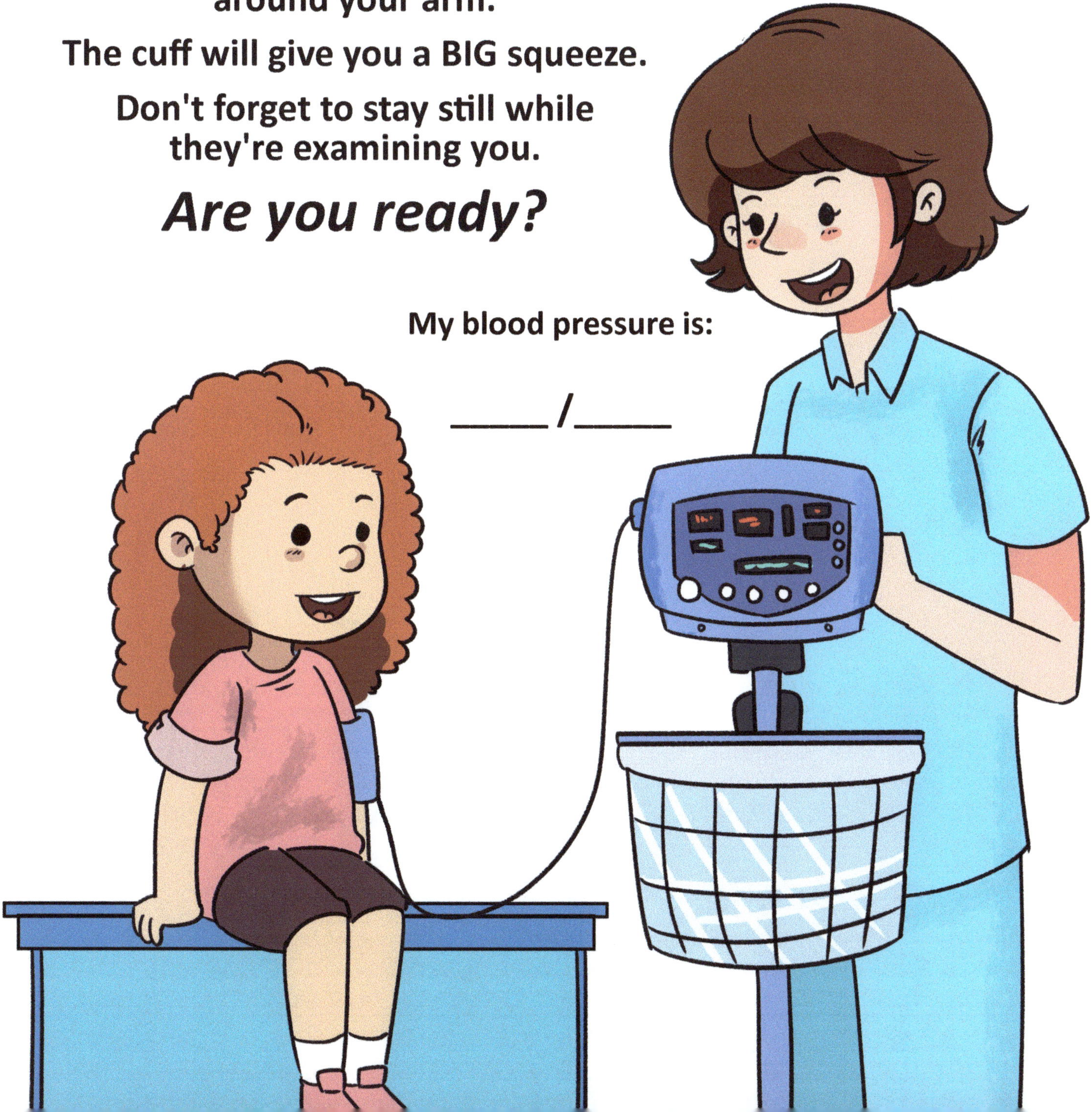

My blood pressure is:

_____ / _____

Your nurse will also check your heart rate, breathing, oxygen level in your blood, and temperature.

My heart rate is: _____ / minute

My breathing is: _____ / minute

My oxygen level is: _____ %

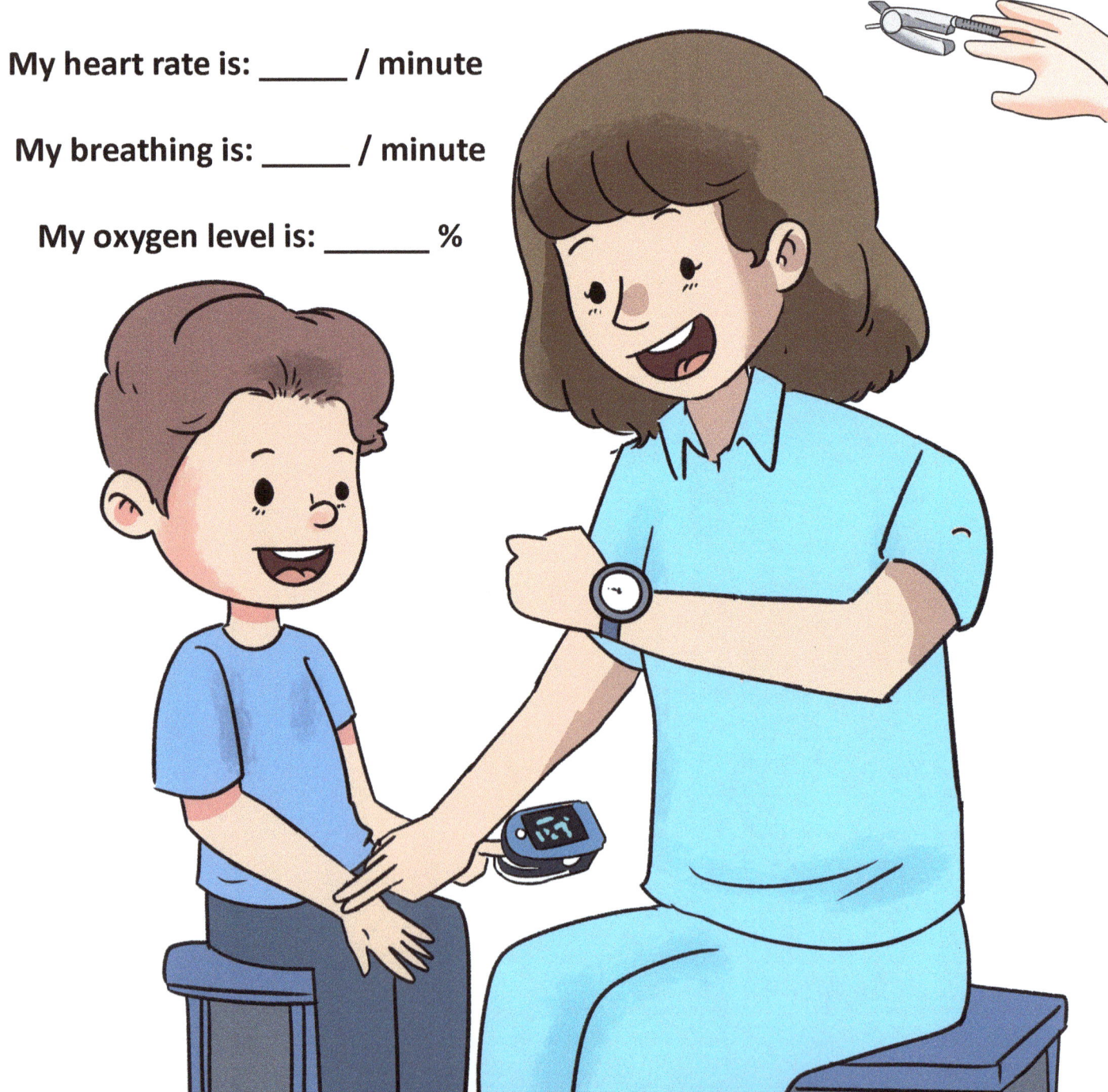

They may even check your vision and hearing to make sure they stay healthy.

My temperature is:
_____

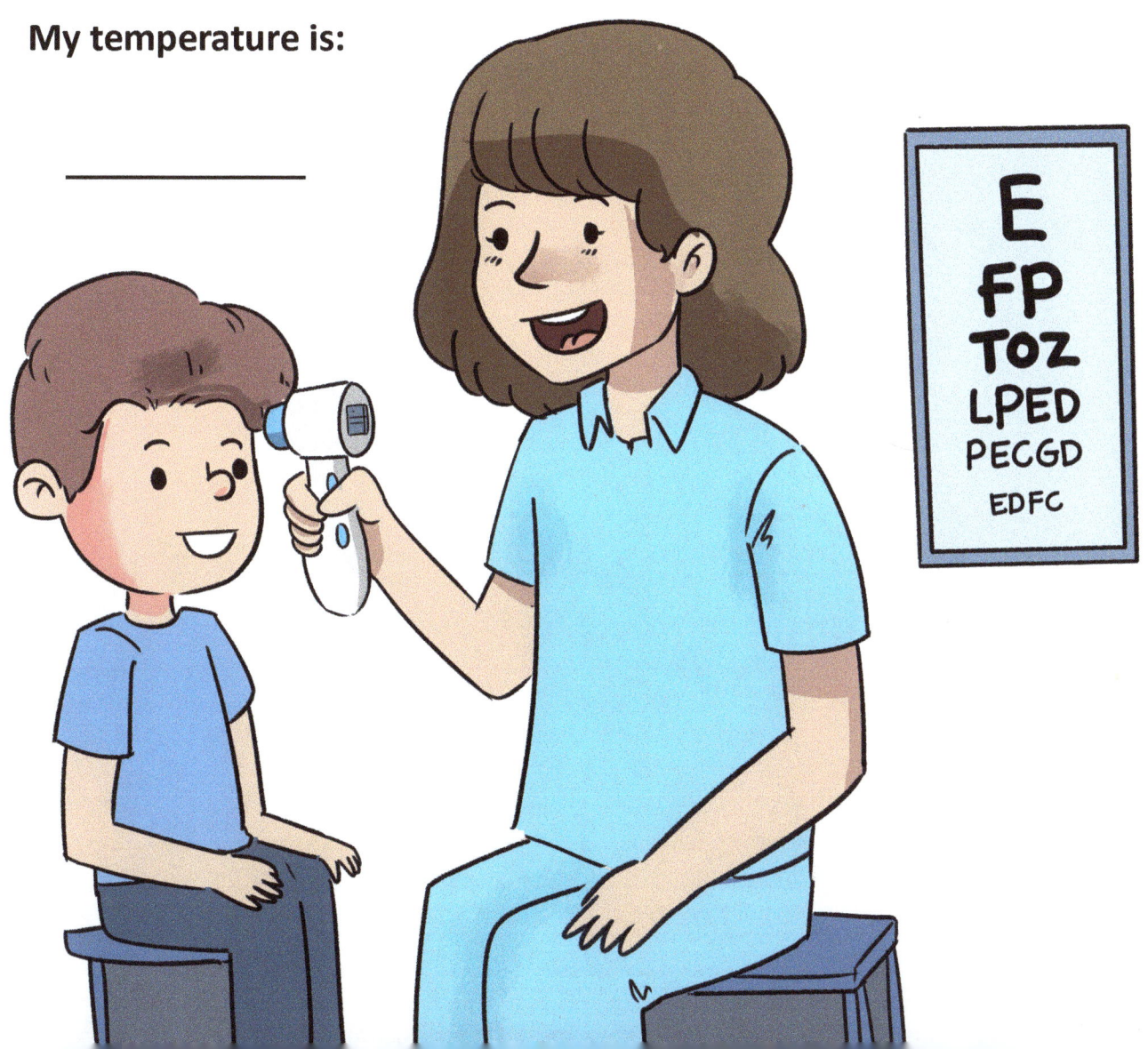

Let's check out the room they have prepared for you.

Can you spot the following in the room?

1) An exam table covered with a long piece of white paper for your protection
2) Special medical tools (flashlights) on the wall
3) A computer monitor
4) A trashcan   5) A box of gloves   6) Some chairs

What are some pictures on the walls in your exam room?

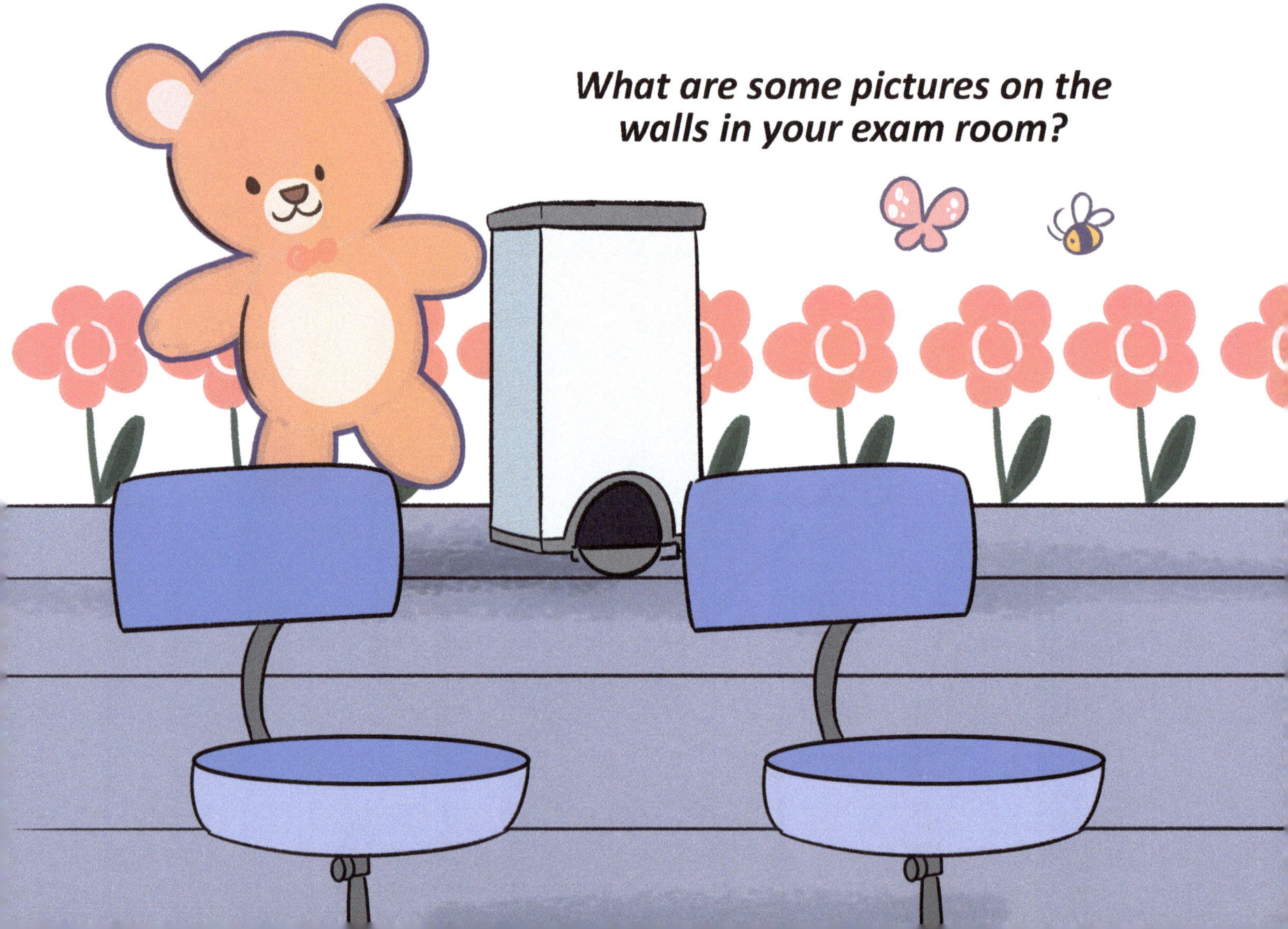

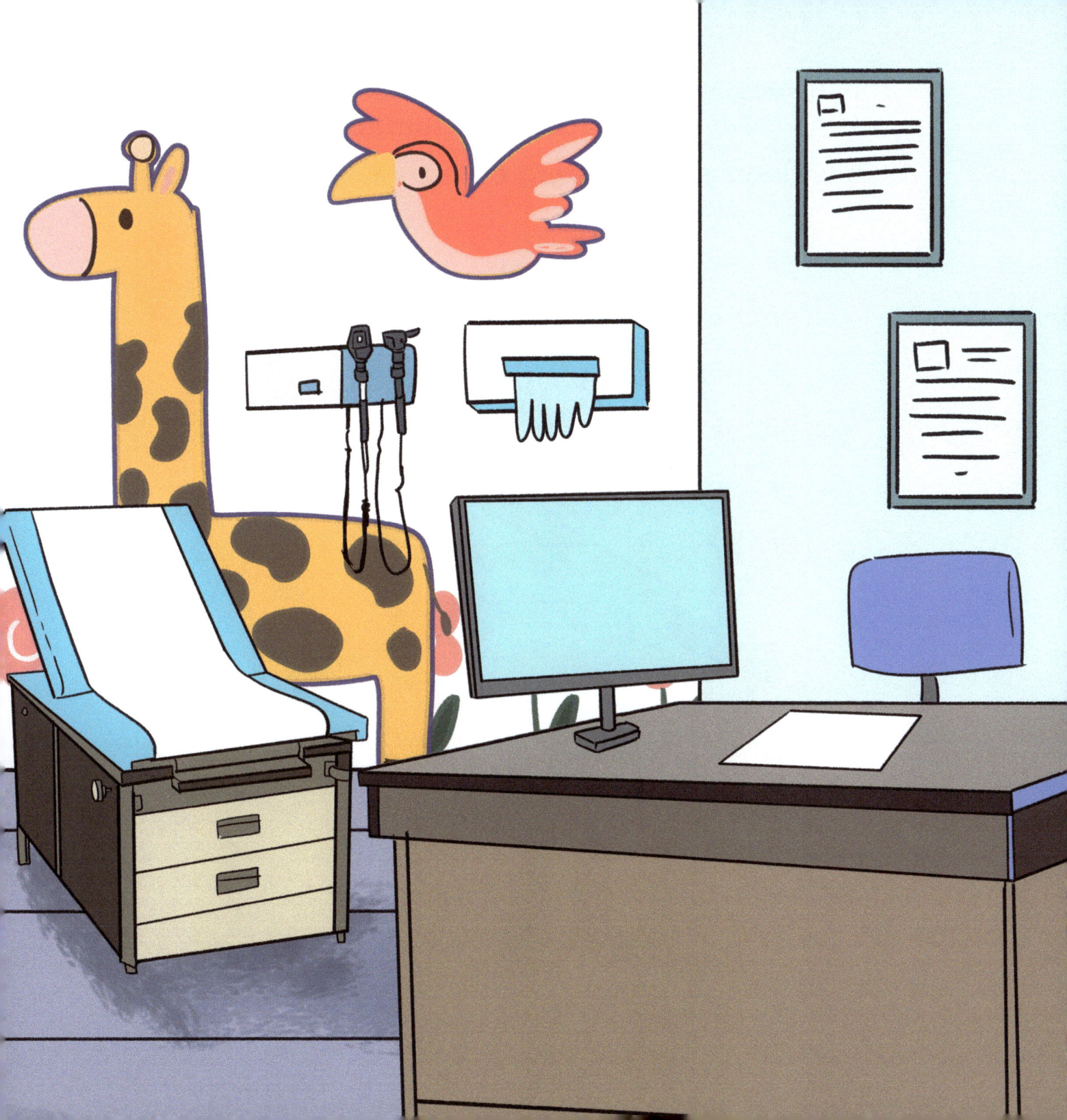

Sometimes, you may need to change into a gown that looks like a backward superhero cape.

Don't worry; your parent or guardian will help you.

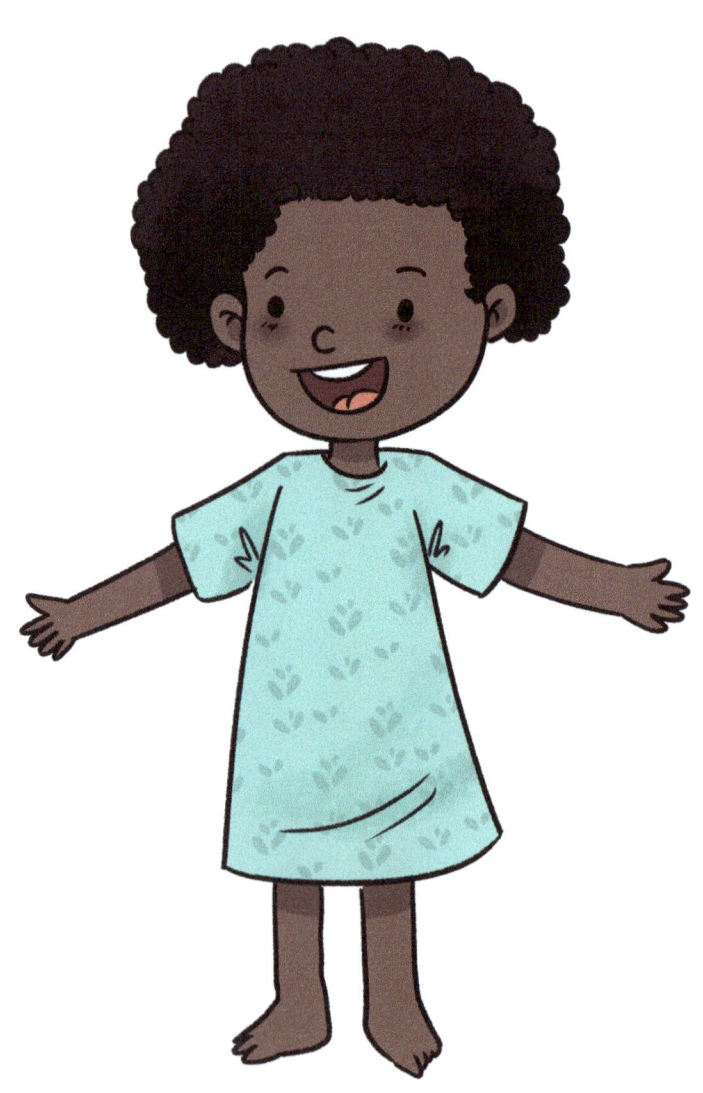

Soon, you'll see your doctor.
Your doctor is friendly, caring, and gentle.

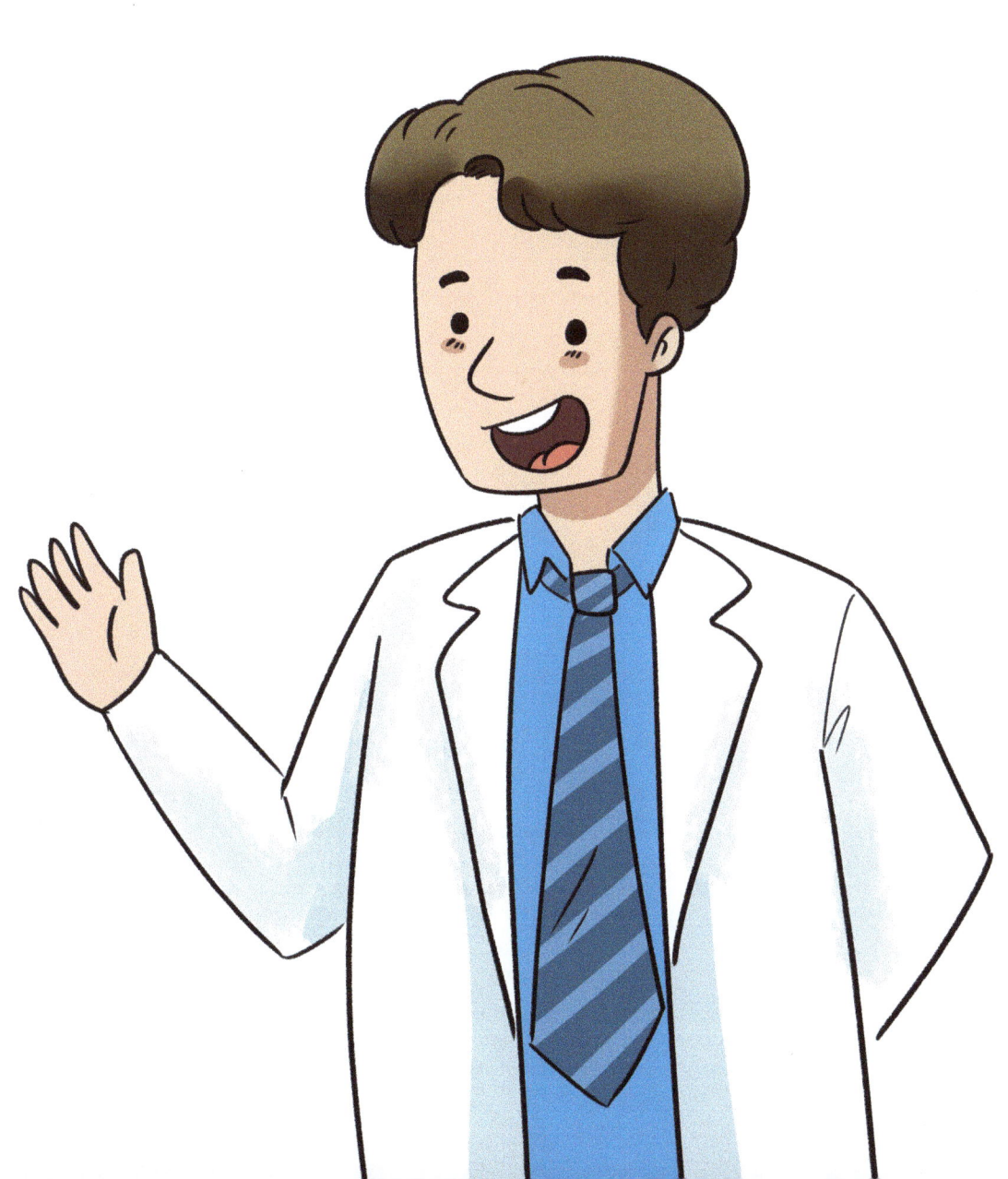

Your parent will talk with your doctor to let them know how you've been doing.

If you have questions for your doctor, don't be afraid to ask.

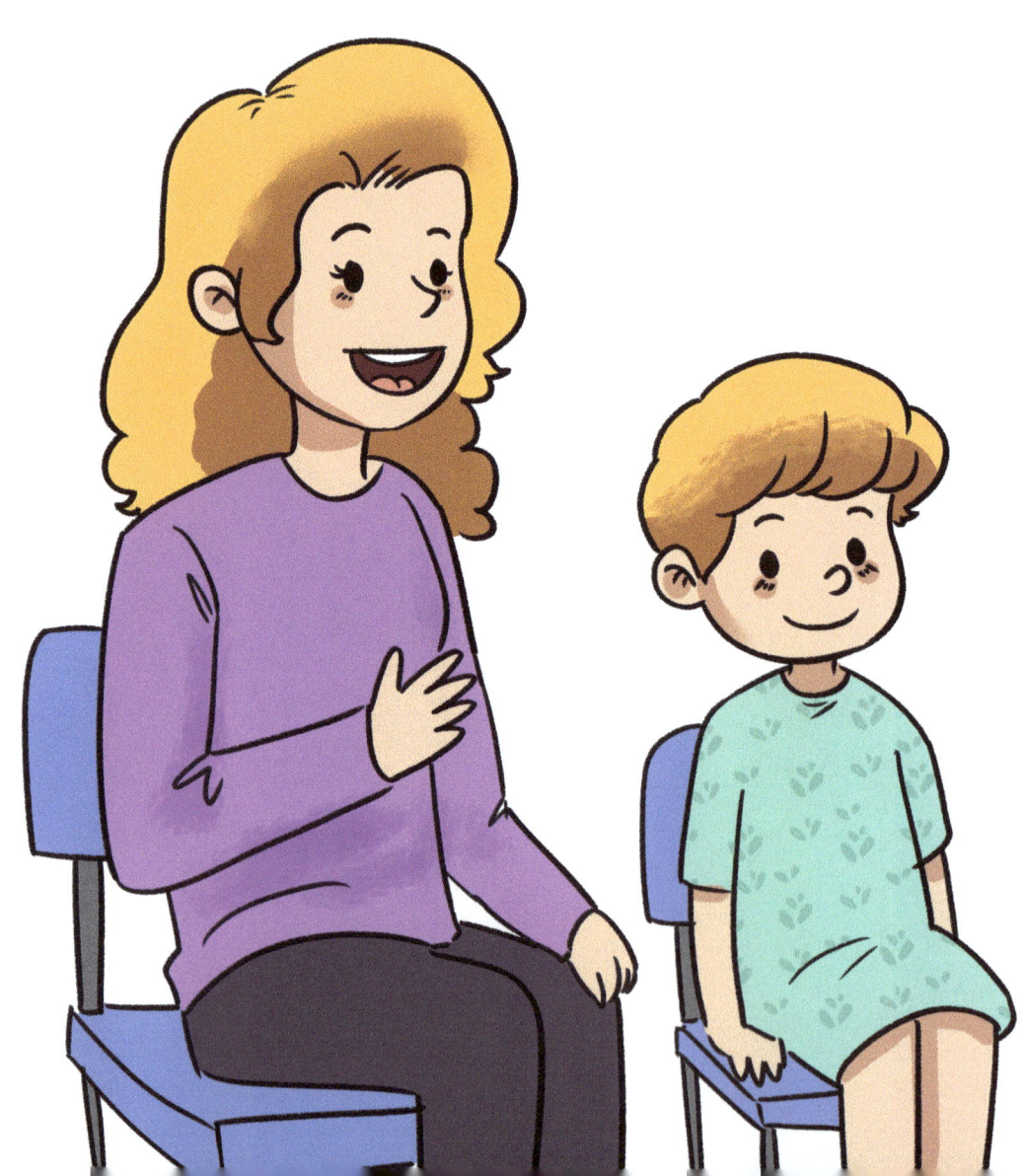

Please write your questions below.

_____

_____

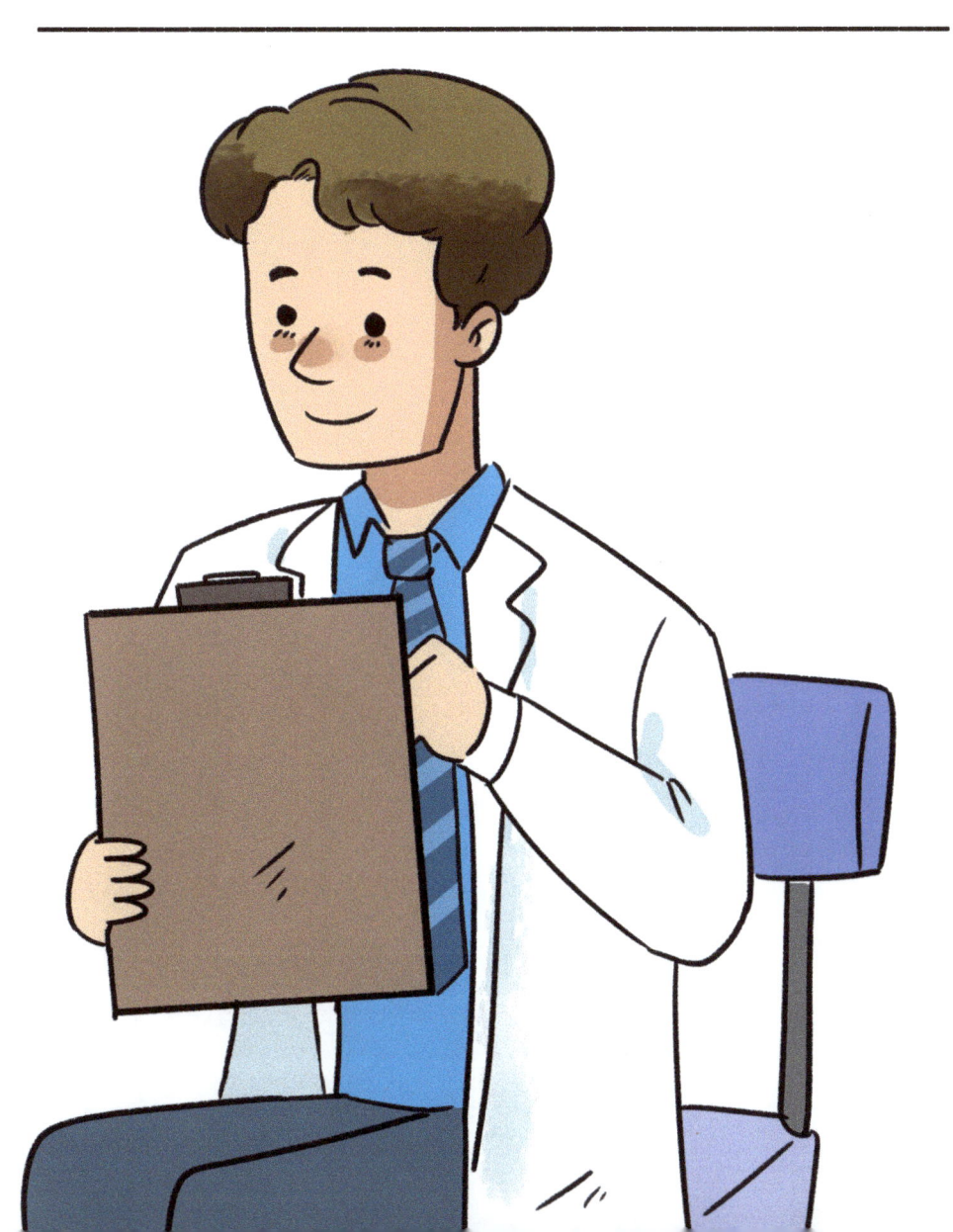

Your doctor will listen to your heart, lungs, and belly with their stethoscope. It may feel a little cold, but it won't hurt.

If you would like to listen, you may ask your doctor if you could borrow their stethoscope.

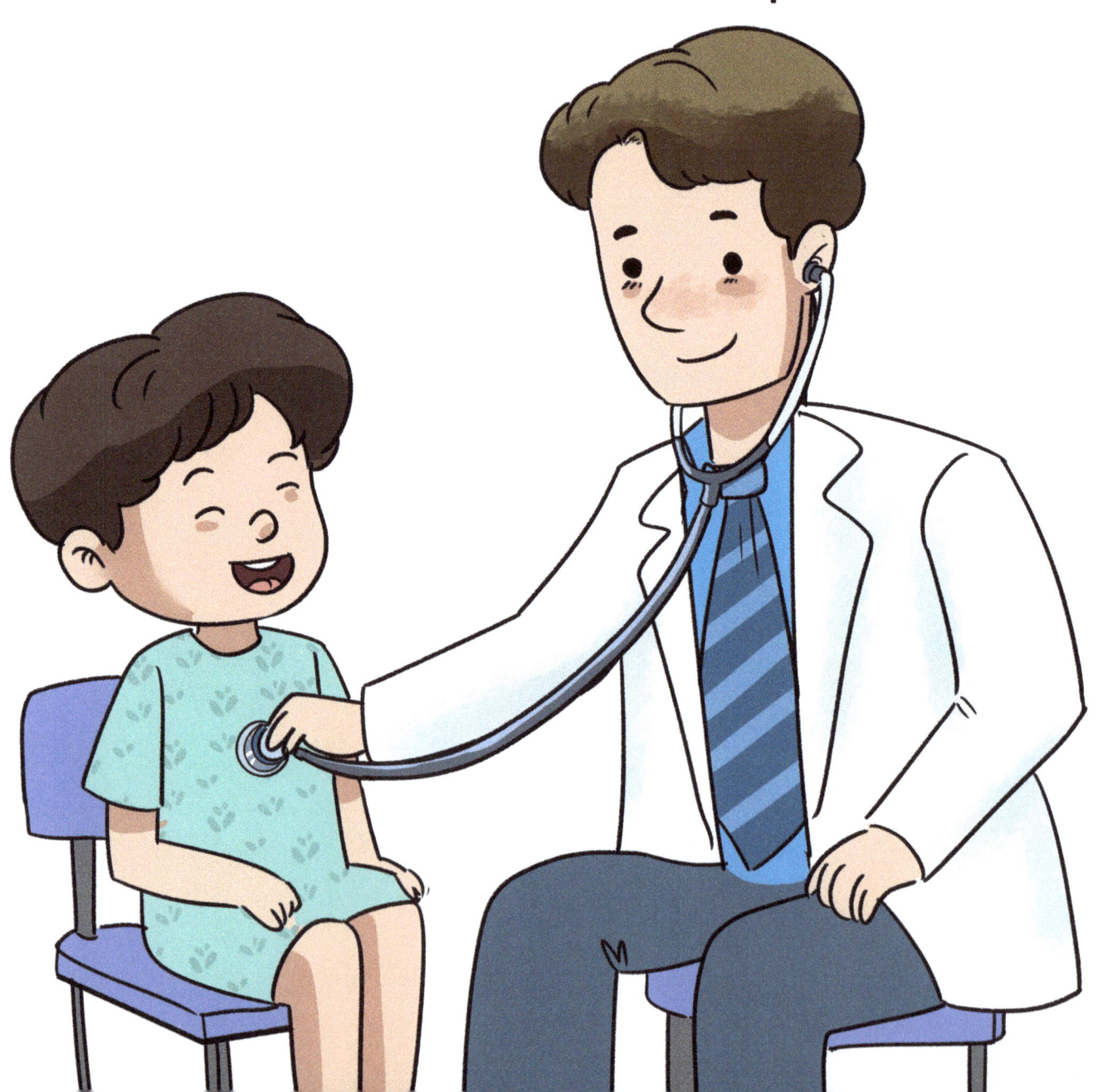

They will also check your eyes, ears, nose, and mouth with their special flashlights.

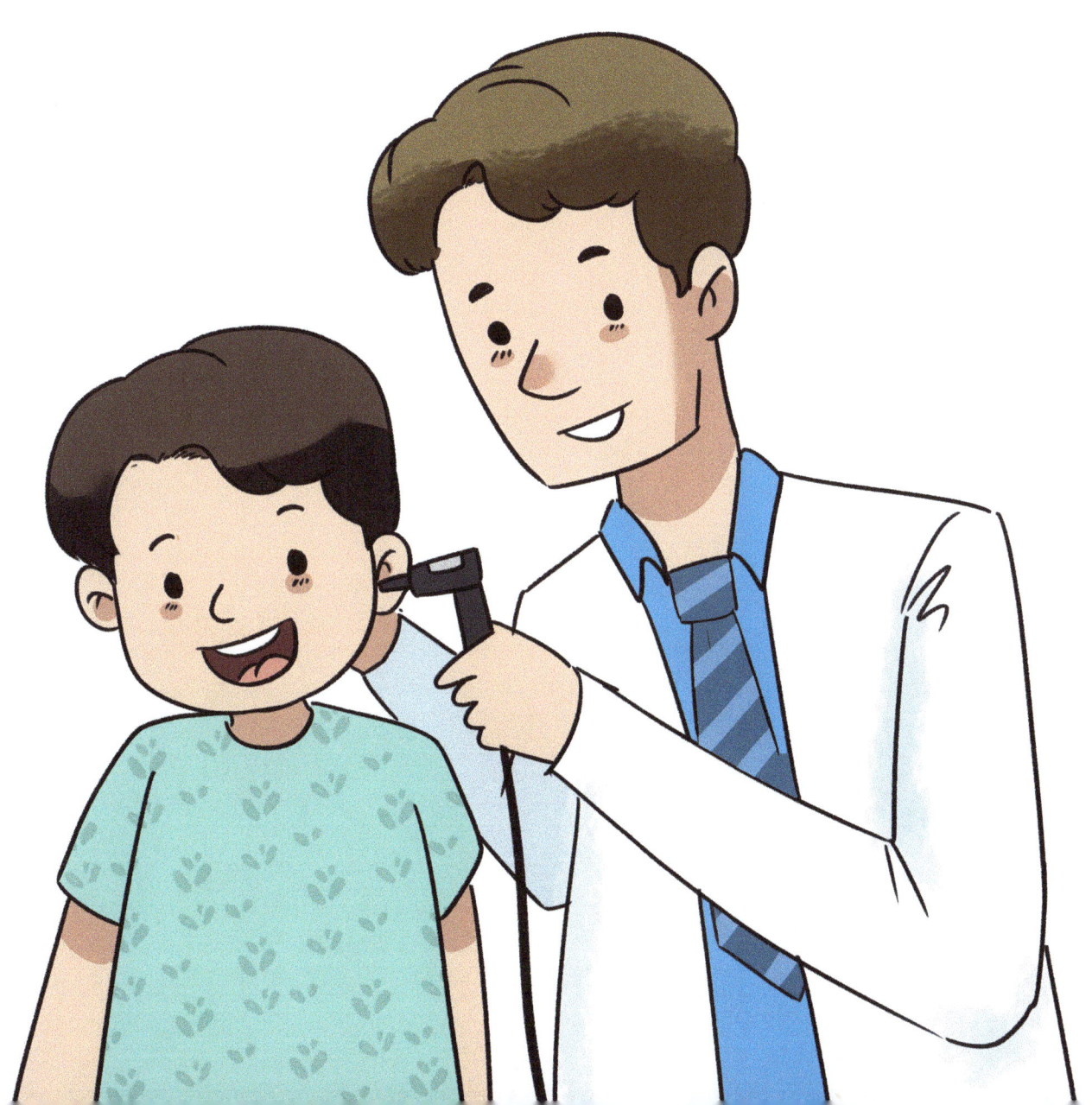

Sometimes, they will use a wooden stick that looks like a popsicle stick to press down on your tongue gently.

Can you say aah or roar like a dinosaur (or bear) and let your doctor look inside your mouth?

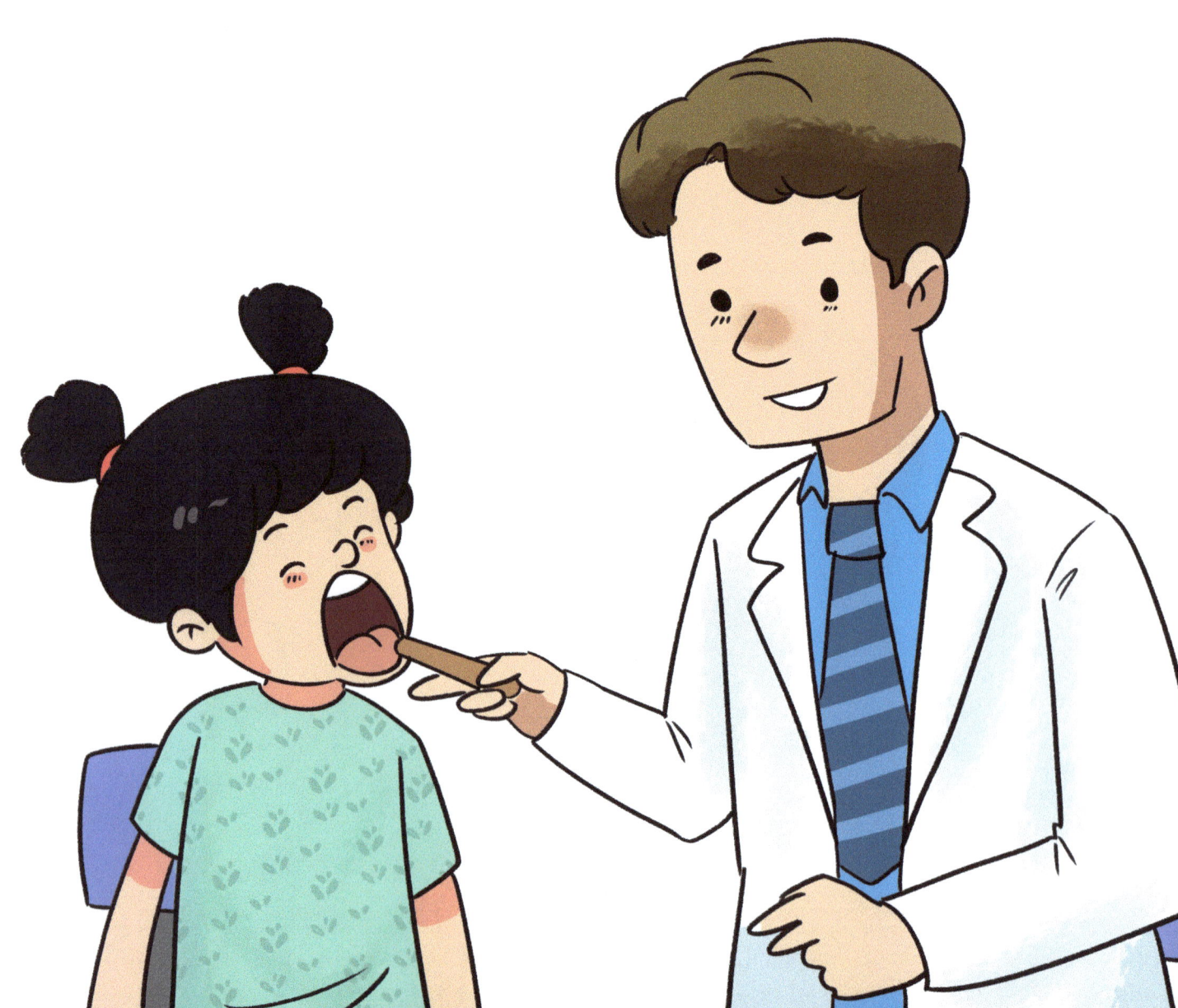

They may even have you touch your nose.

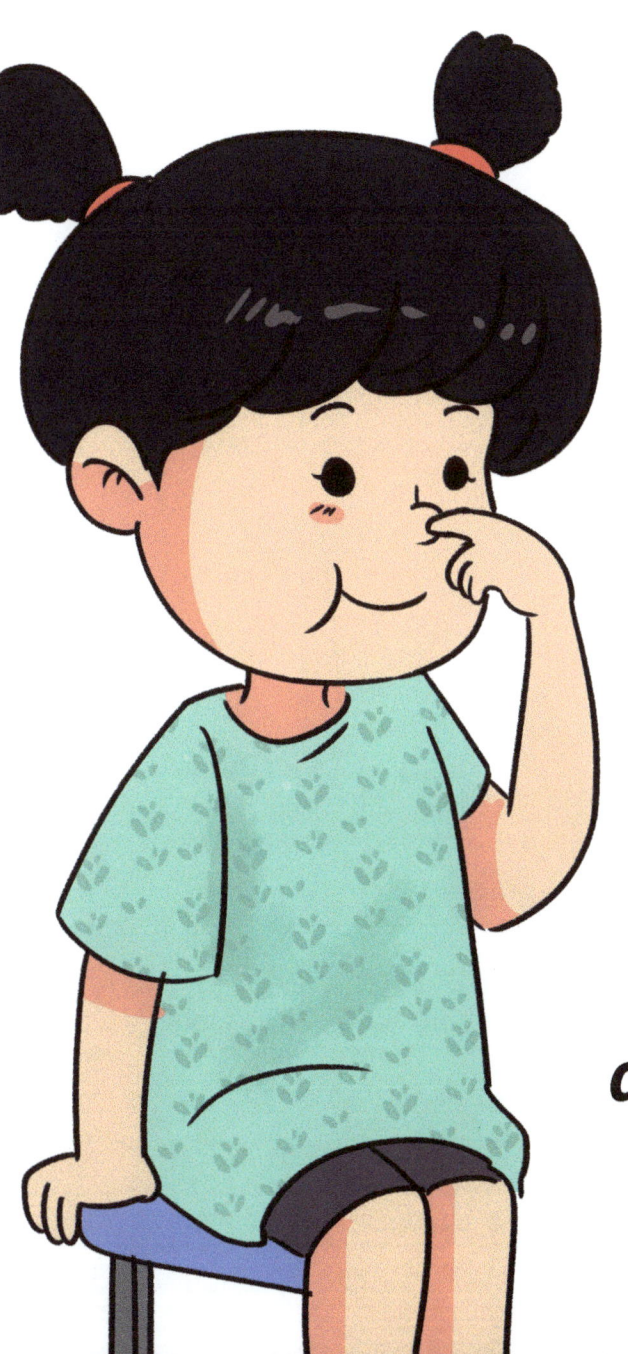

Are you able to touch your nose with your left pointer finger (also called index finger)?

How about with your right pointer finger?

You are doing great!

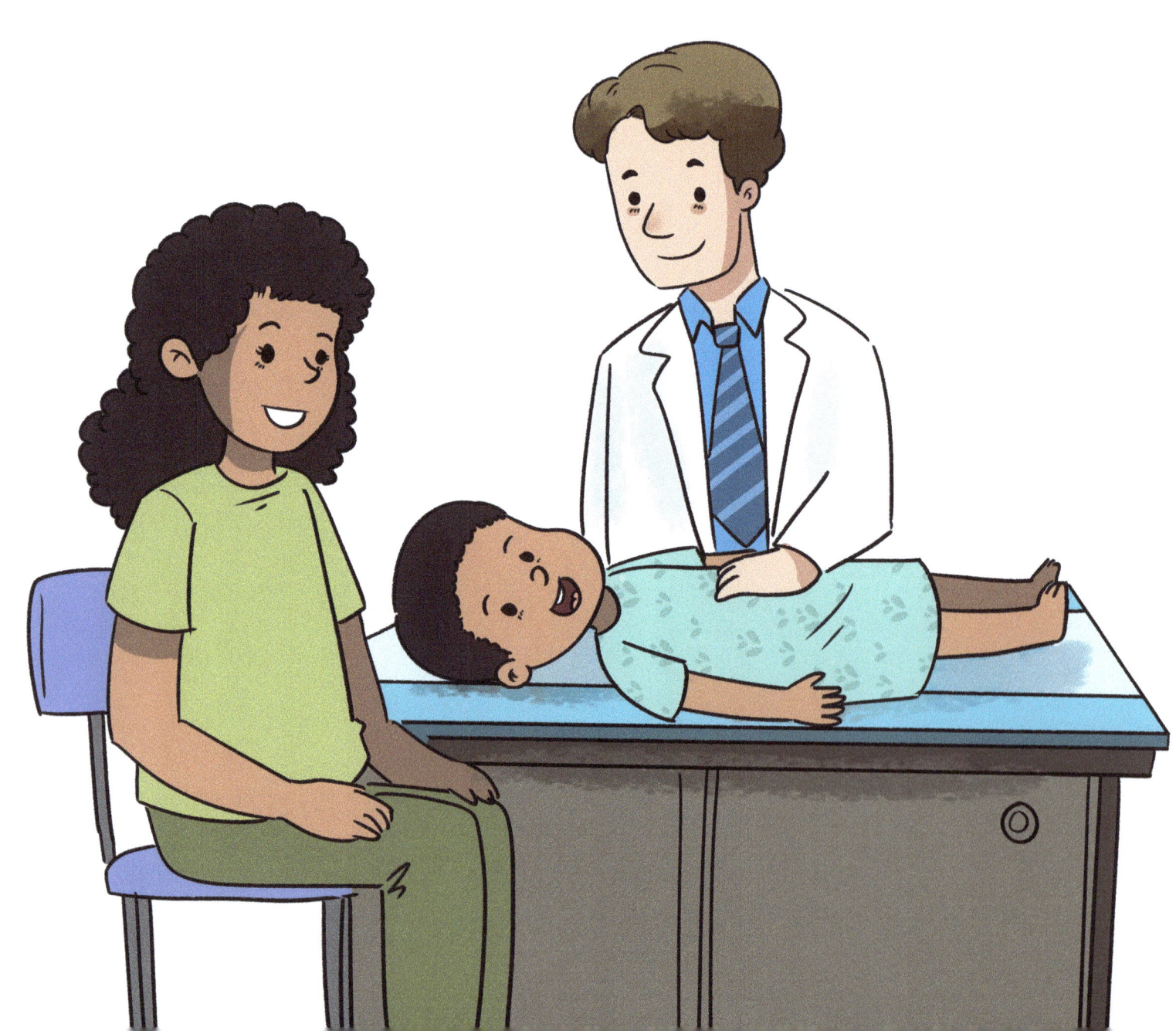

Your doctor may gently press on your chin, neck, and belly to make sure your body on the inside is growing healthy.

They may even check the bottom of your feet.

Don't worry, your parent will stay with you the whole time to make sure you are safe.

If anything bothers you, let your doctor know.

Some kids get ticklish when the doctor examines their body.

Are you ticklish?

Circle your answer: Yes or No

Who wiggles more when tickled?
You or a worm?

Do you think you can stay still for a little while?

Maybe you can try bending your knees to see if that helps.

Your doctor may even check your reflexes (how fast you react without thinking about it) **by gently tapping below your knees and on your arms with a reflex hammer made out of rubber.**

Relax your body and let the reflex hammer do its job.

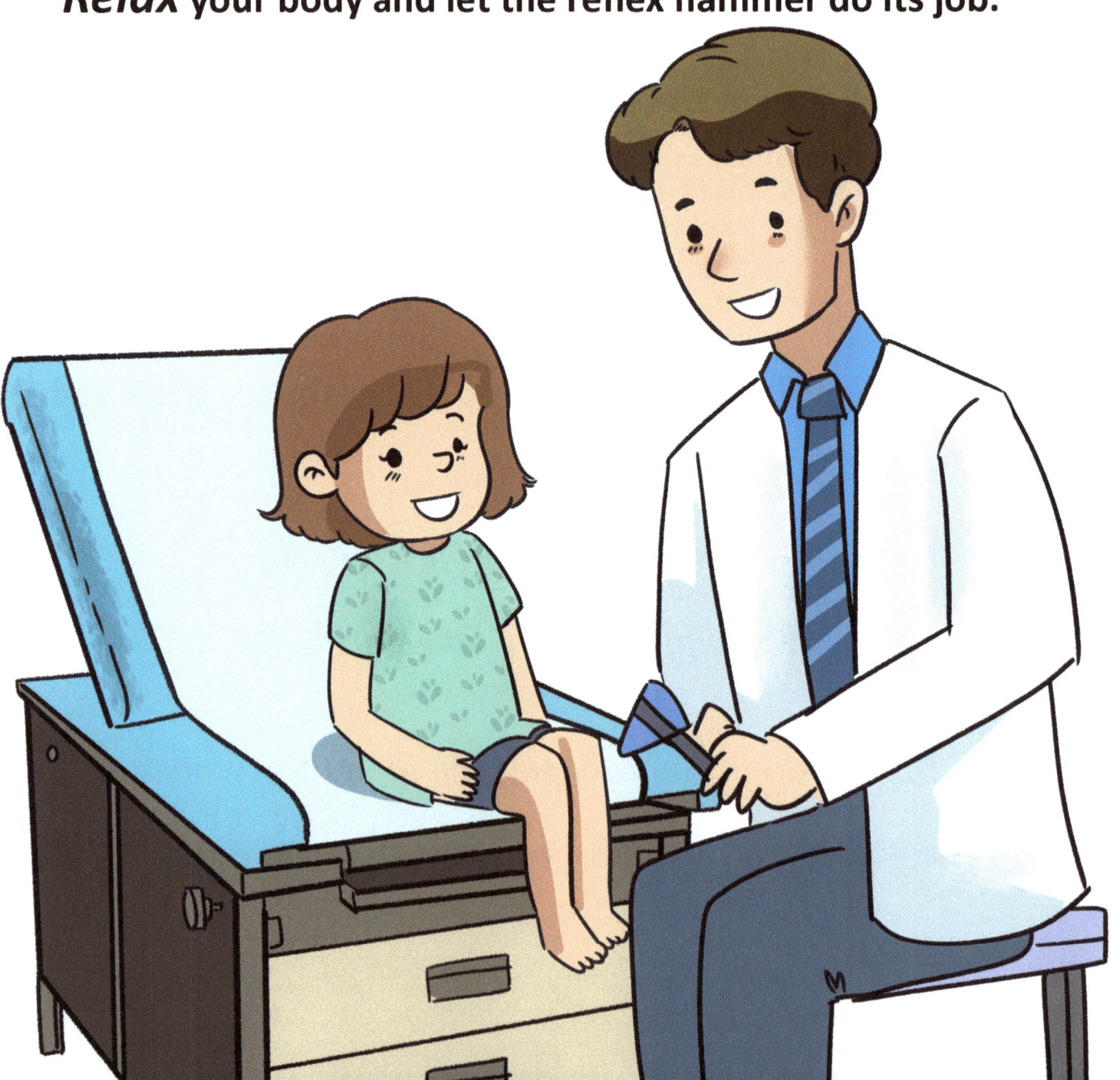

Do you know what happens when the reflex hammer gently taps your knees?

How did it make you feel?

Did it make you giggle?

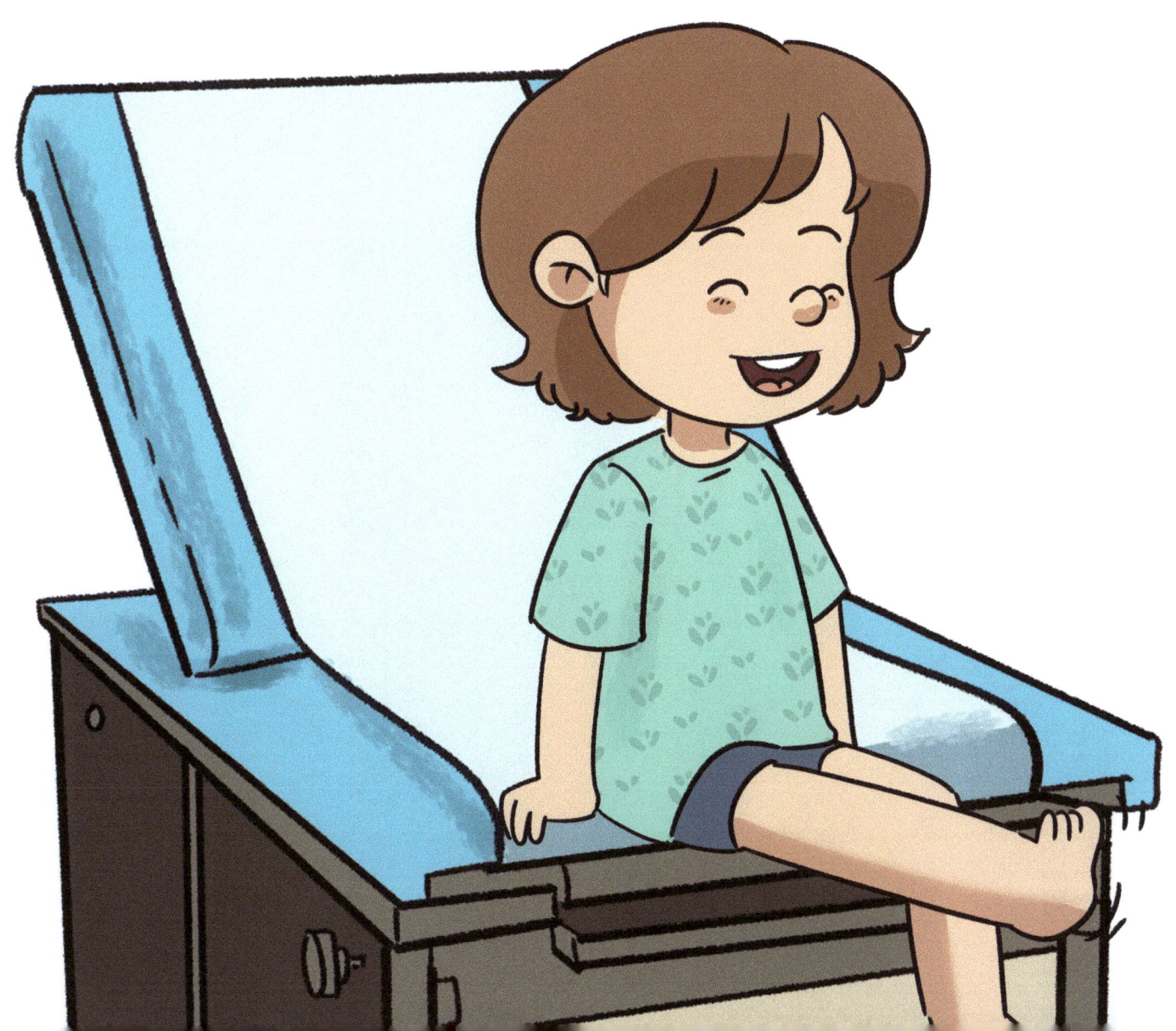

Your doctor may check your spine and joints like your shoulders, elbows, wrists, hips, knees and ankles.

They may also check your private parts to make sure they are also growing healthy.

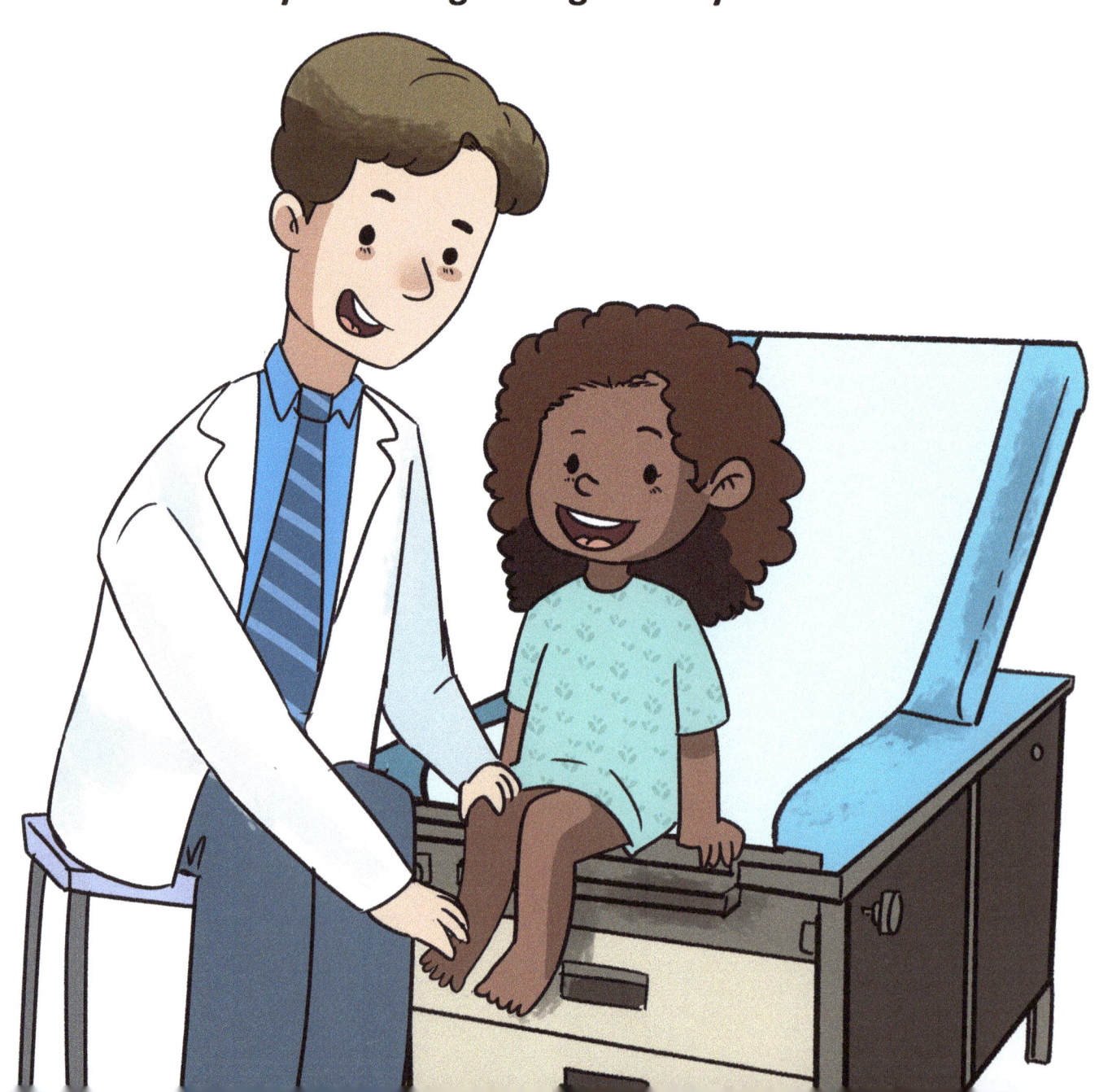

Don't worry, your parent will stay with you the whole time to make sure you are safe.

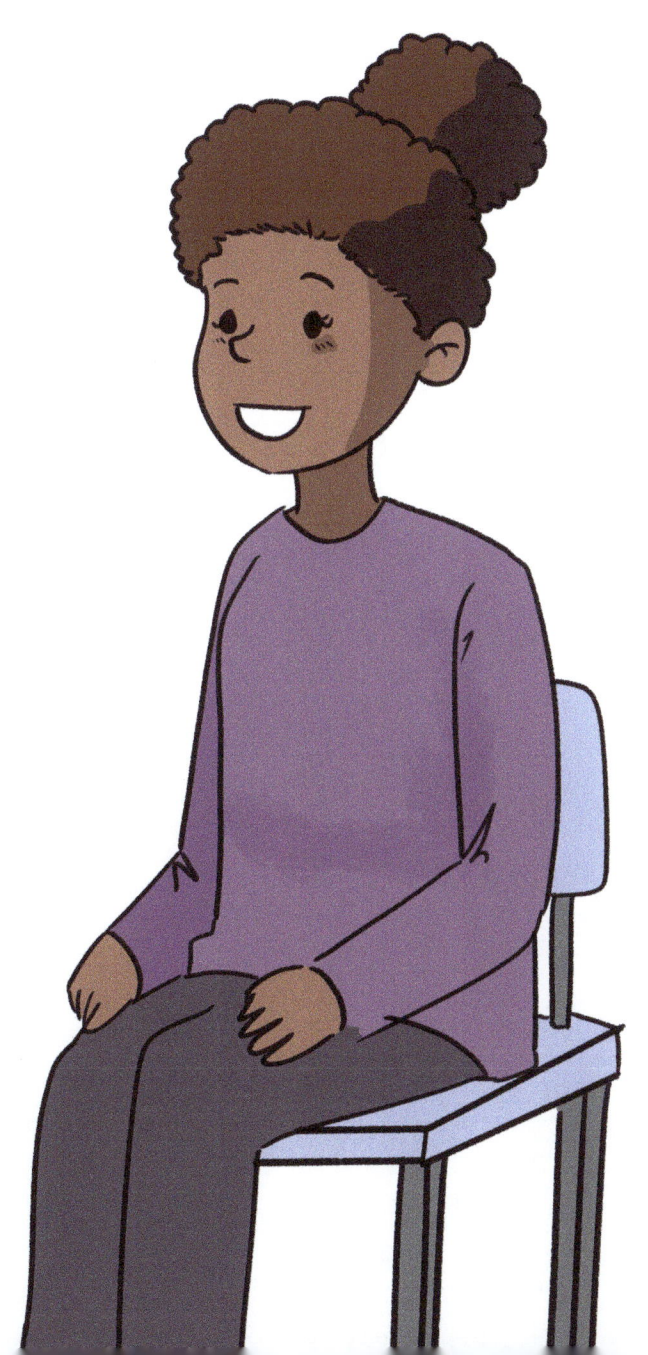

After your doctor checks you from head to toe and tells you everything is good, your adventure at the doctor's office is almost over.

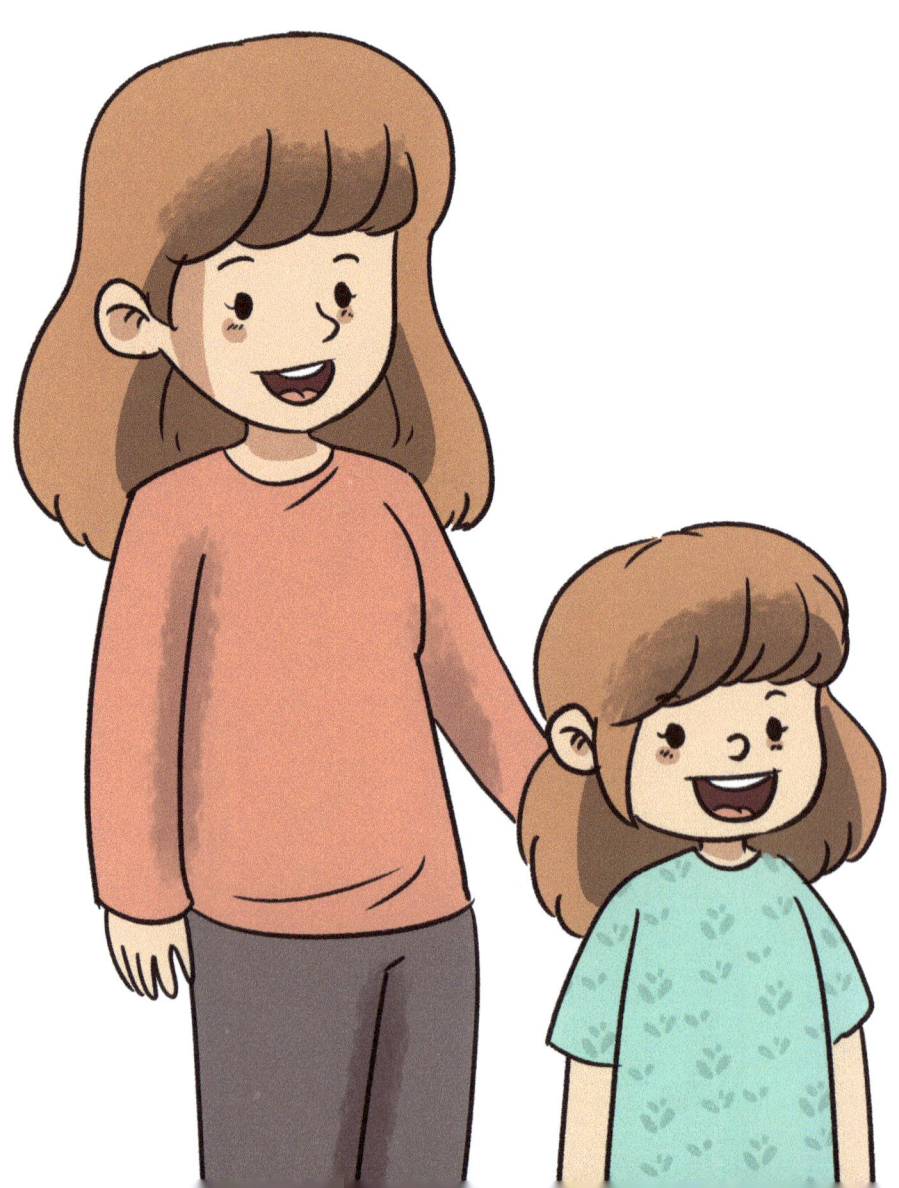

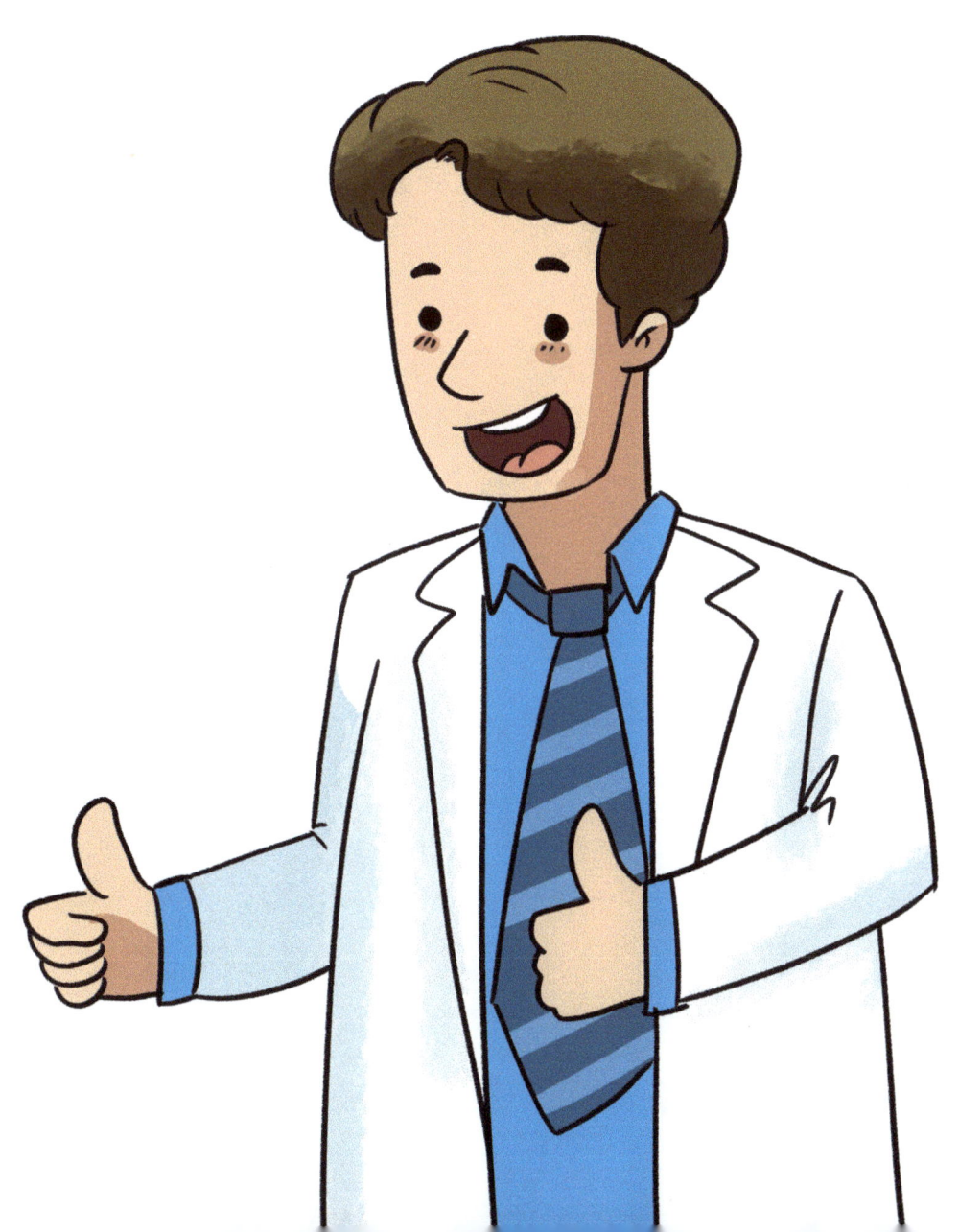

Sometimes, you may need to get a shot. It feels like a quick, tiny poke.

Take a deep breath in and out.

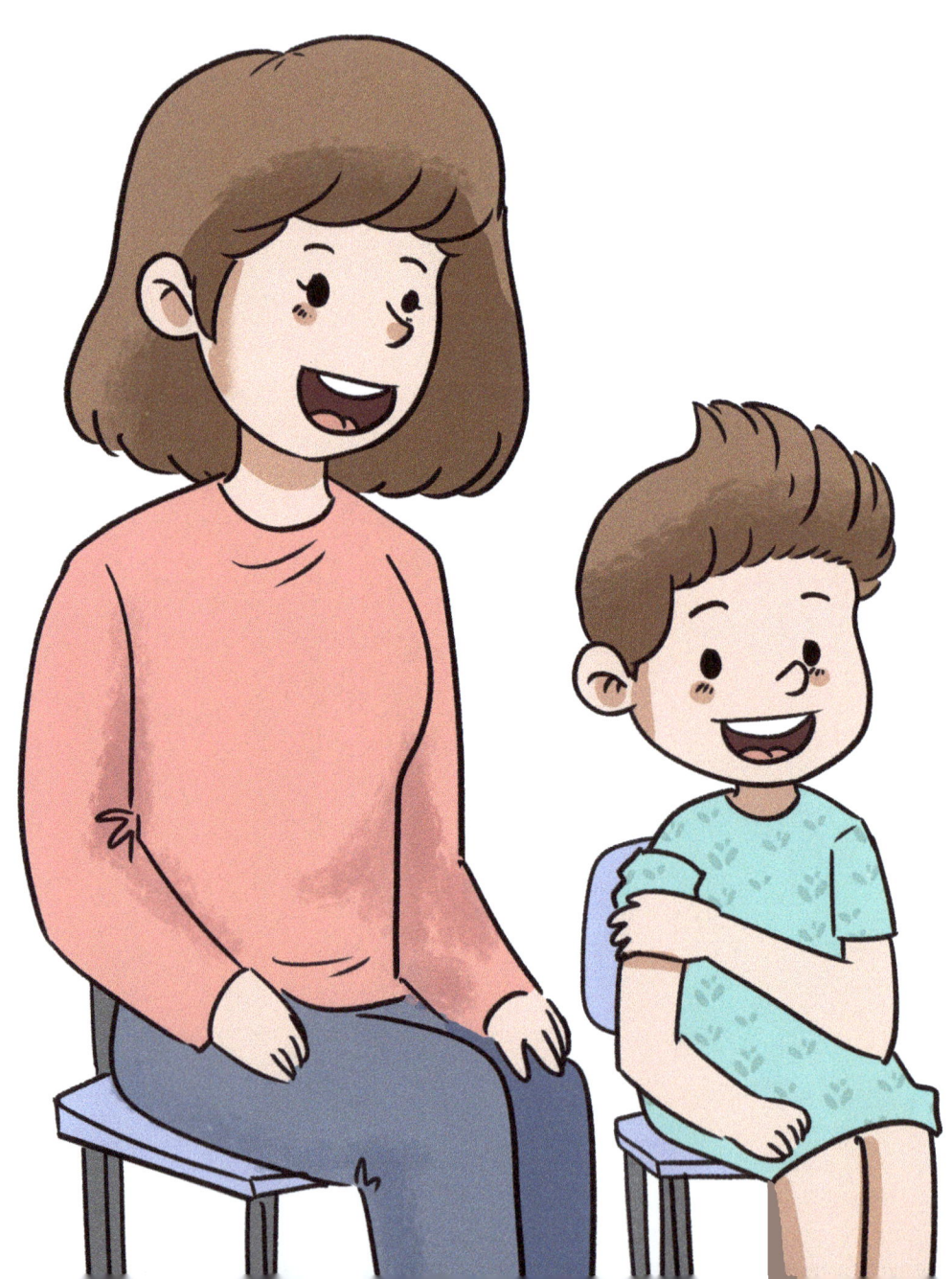

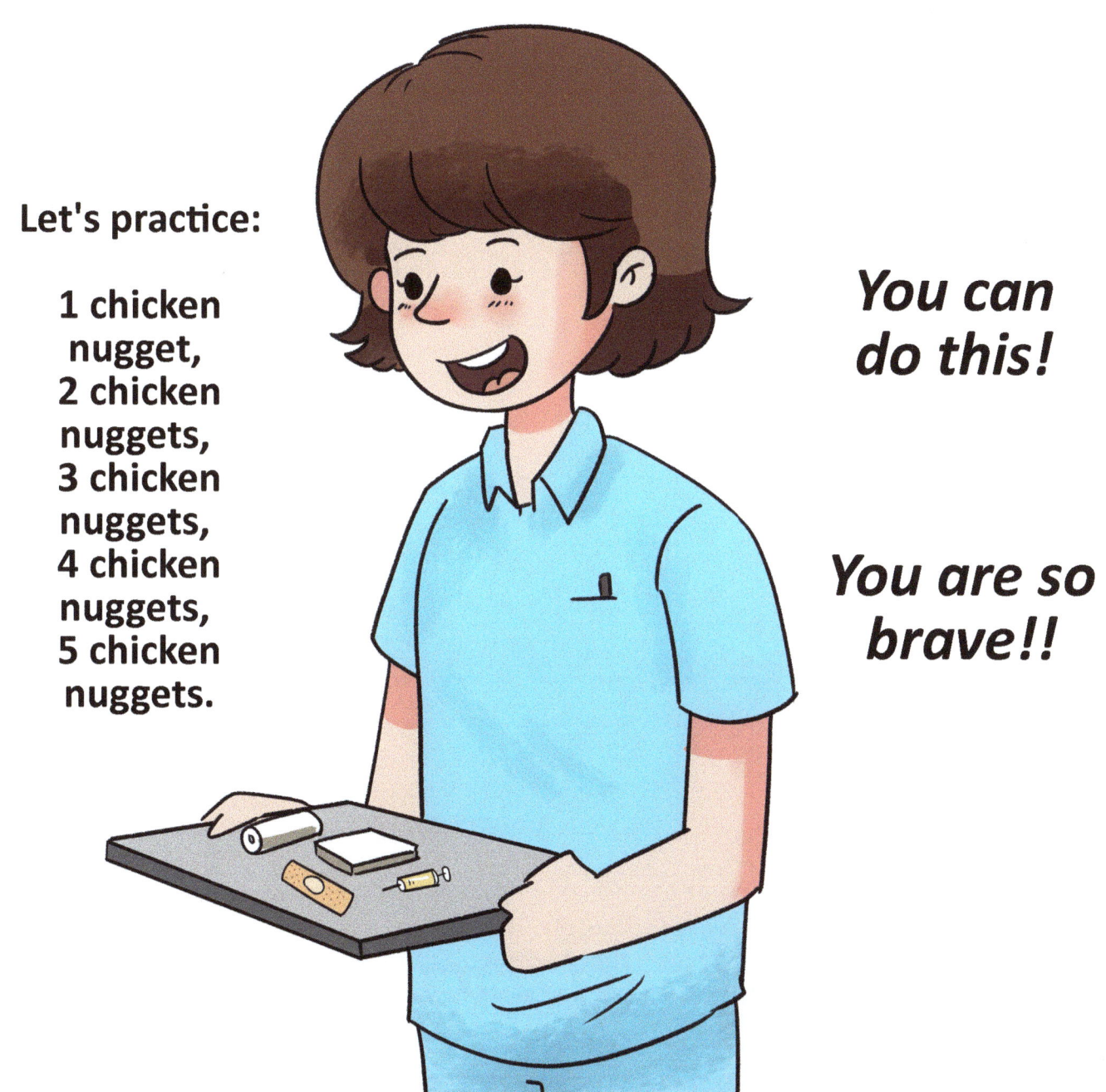

What will you do after your doctor's visit?

A party? A celebration?

What's your favorite way to celebrate?

Draw or write your party plan below.

You did it! Excellent job!

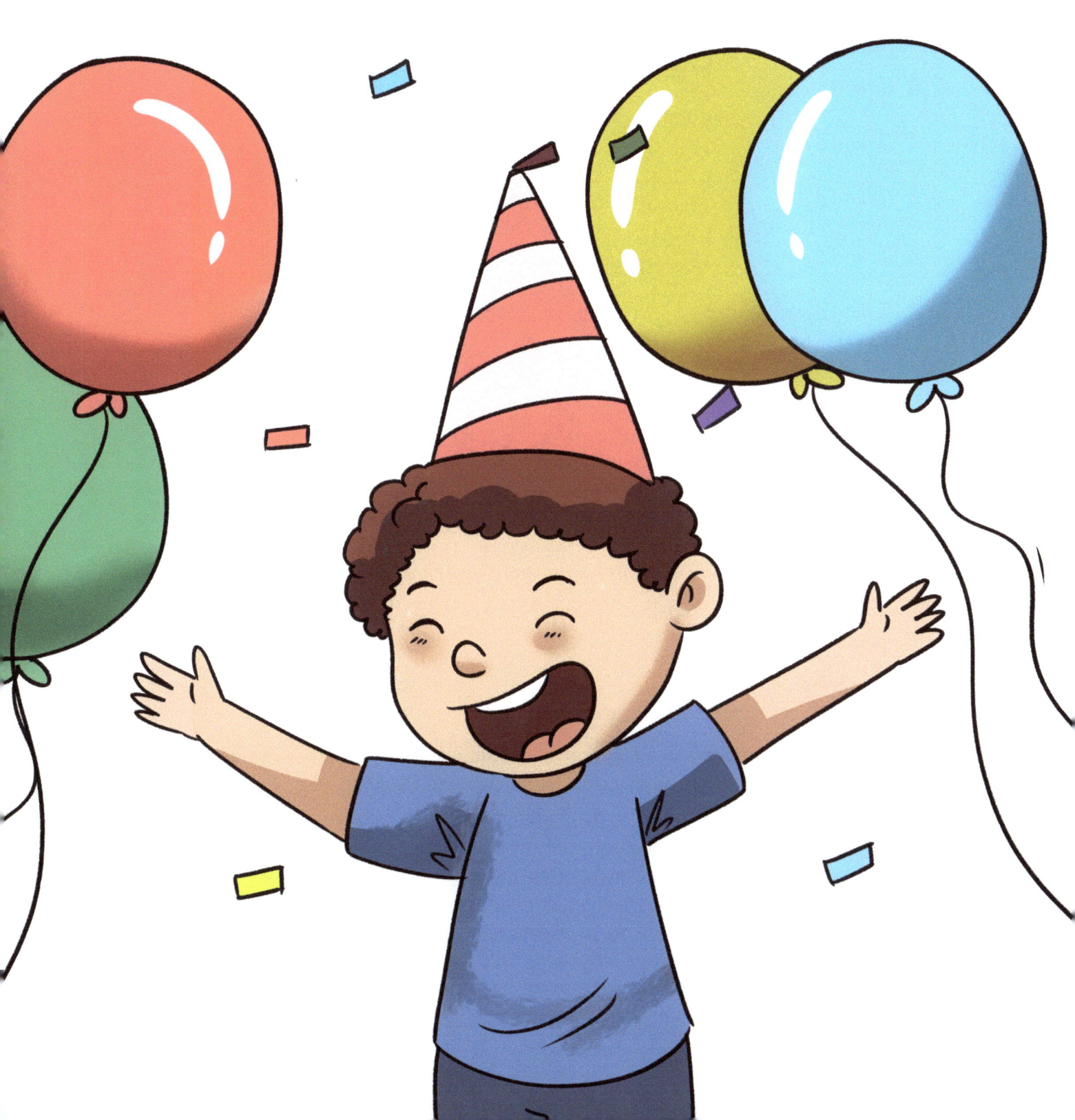

Did this picture book help your child in some way?
If so, I would love to hear about it!

www.amazon.com/gp/product-review/B0DHWFNR4Z

For other book titles, please visit:

www.fzwbooks.com

Connect with the Author

email: books@fzwbooks.com
facebook/instagram: @FZWbooks

Disclaimer

Please note that the illustrations are not drawn to scale.

This book is written for informational, educational, and personal growth purposes and should not be used as a substitute for medical advice.

Please consult your child's doctor if they need medical attention and to ensure the information in this book pertains to your child's medical condition and needs. I cannot guarantee what your child experiences is exactly what is being discussed in this book.

The author and the publisher are not responsible, either directly or indirectly, for any damages, monetary losses, or reparations due to information in this book. By reading this book, the readers agree not to hold the author and the publisher responsible for any losses as a result of any errors, inaccuracies, or omissions in this book.

Please keep in mind that your child's experience depends on the location, the facility, their medical condition, and the healthcare team. Please use this book in conjunction with your child's doctor's advice. Thank you.

About the Author

Dr. Fei Zheng-Ward is a clinical anesthesiologist who understands the apprehension patients (both adults and children) may have surrounding their upcoming surgery. Her goal in her medical books is to bring useful information to patients so they have a better understanding and appreciation of what happens leading up to, during, and after surgery. She wants readers to be more empowered to make informed decisions and to feel more at ease with their surgery.

As a practicing physician, she takes pride in being respected for her attention to detail, commitment to providing compassionate and personalized patient care, and strong presence in patient advocacy in the perioperative period for each of her patients. She understands the importance of physical and emotional well-being and advocates for patient autonomy.

Her other children's books aim to bring laughter into your family, encourage children to be more helpful at home, and inspire a love of reading.

She is an award-winning author for her book titled **What to Expect and How to Prepare for Your Surgery**.

More about Dr. Fei Zheng-Ward:

- Board Certified Anesthesiologist

- Anesthesiology Residency Training at The Johns Hopkins Hospital in Baltimore, MD

- Master in Public Health (MPH) degree from Dartmouth Medical School in Hanover, NH

Books by the author

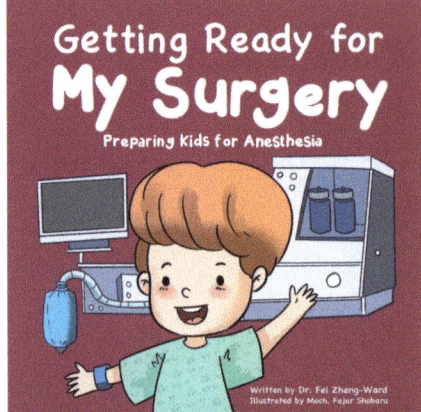
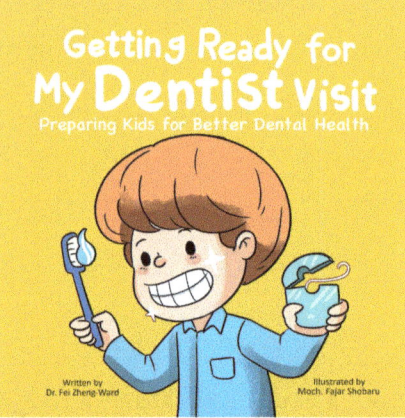
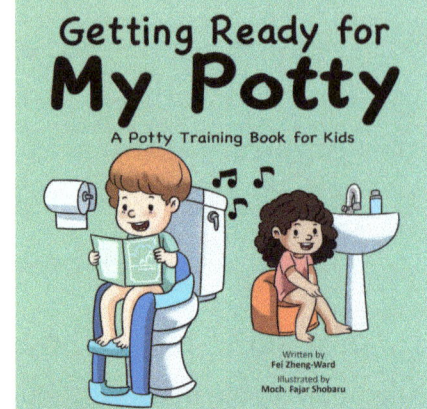
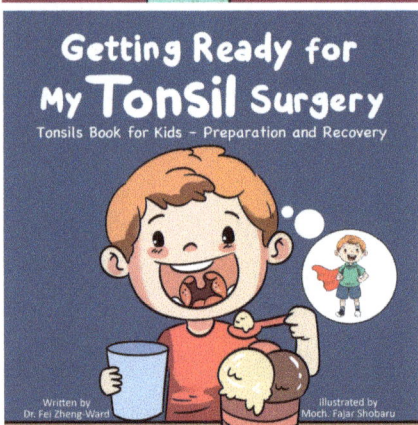
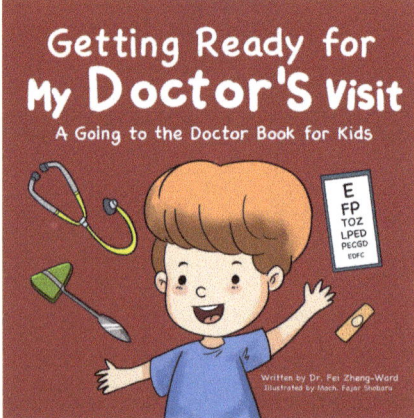
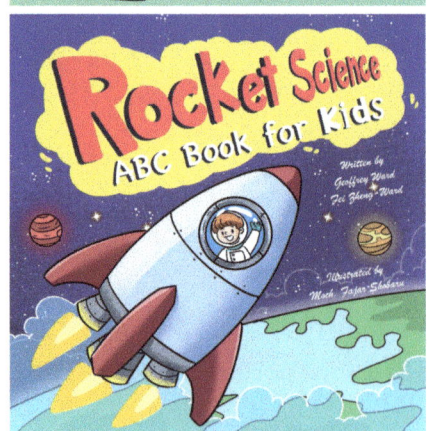
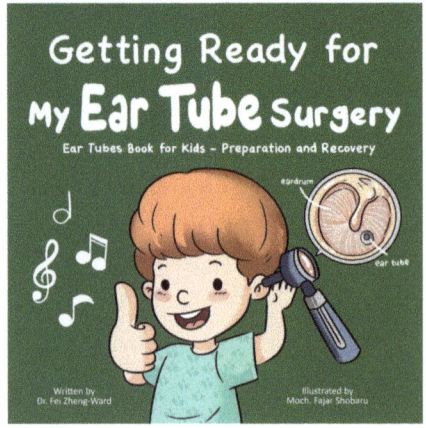
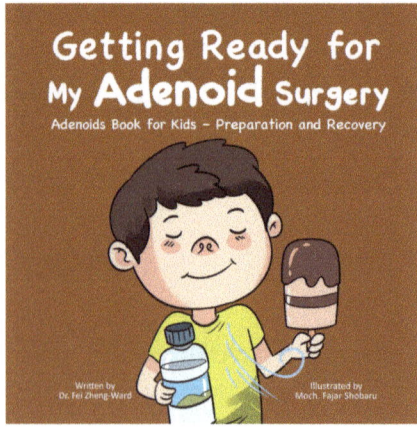
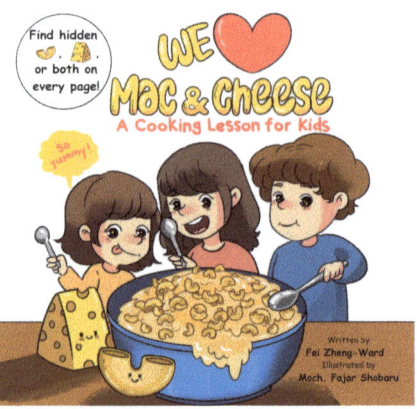

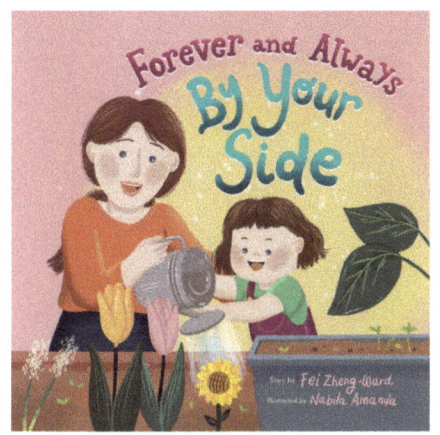
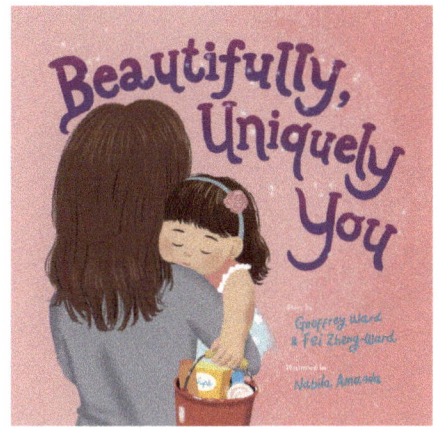
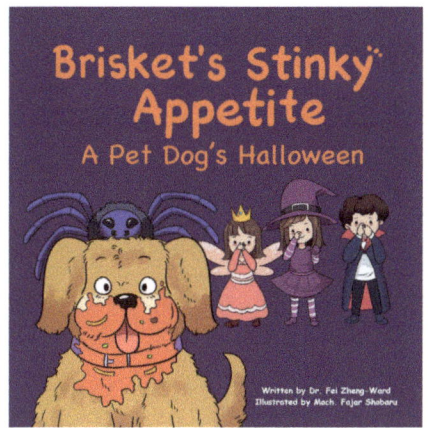
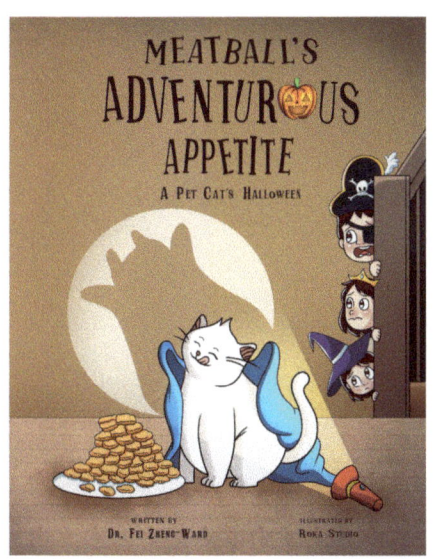
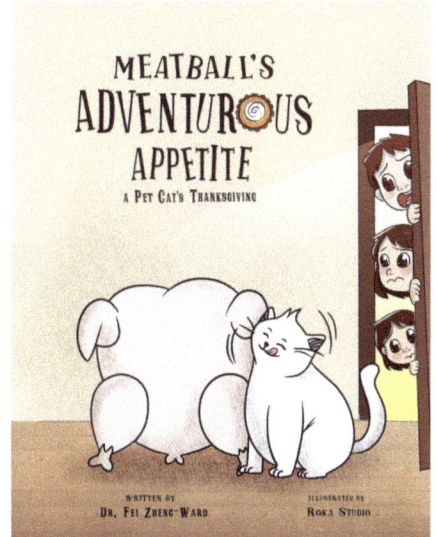
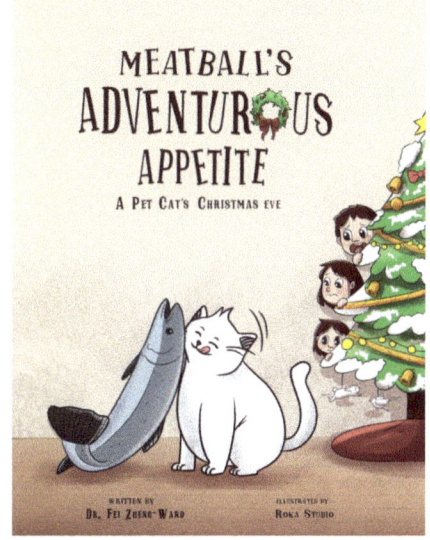
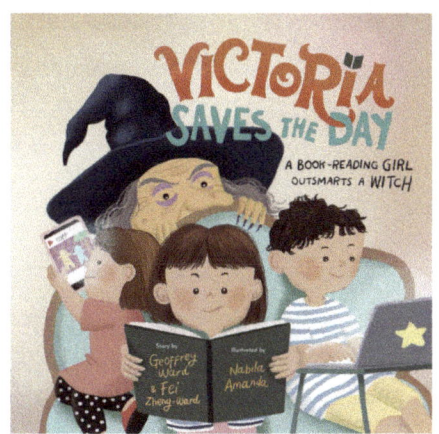
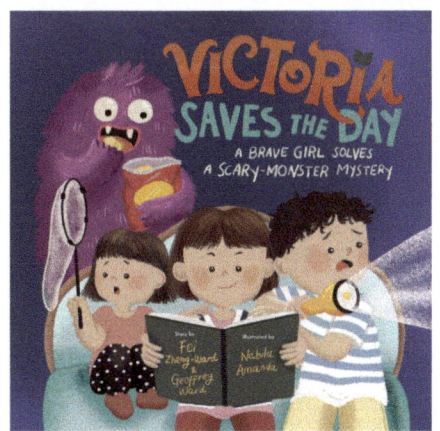
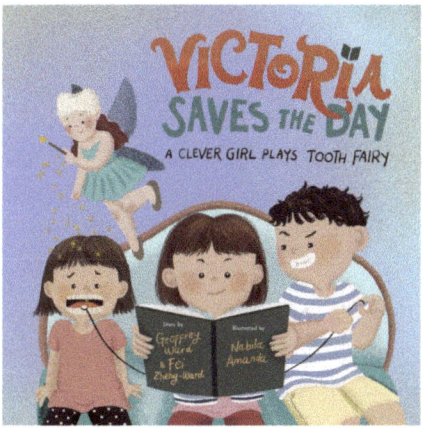